The Paraprofessional in Home Health and Long-Term Care

This book is printed on recycled paper.

The Paraprofessional in Home Health and Long-Term Care

Training Modules for Working with Older Adults

by

Ellen Cervantes, M.S.W.

Jeanne Heid-Grubman, L.S.W.

and

Charlotte K. Schuerman, L.C.S.W.

The Center for Applied Gerontology
Chicago

HEALTH PROFESSIONS PRESS

Baltimore · London · Toronto · Sydney

Health Professions Press, Inc.
Post Office Box 10624
Baltimore, Maryland 21285-0624

Typeset by Maple-Vail Composition Services, Binghamton, New York.
Manufactured in the United States of America by The Maple Press Company, Binghamton, New York.

Library of Congress Cataloging-in-Publication Data

Cervantes, Ellen.

The paraprofessional in home health and long-term care: training modules for working with older adults / by Ellen Cervantes, Jeanne Heid-Grubman, Charlotte Schuerman.

p. cm.

Includes bibliographical references and index.

ISBN 1-878812-25-4

1. Geriatric nursing. 2. Home health aides. 3. Long-term care of the sick. I. Heid-Grubman, Jeanne. II. Schuerman, Charlotte. III. Title.

RC954.C43 1995

610.73′65–dc20 95-11564

CIP

British Library Cataloguing-in-Publication data are available from the British Library.

Contents

List of Tables and Figures vii
List of Activities xi
About the Authors xiii
Foreword *Wendy Lustbader* xv
Preface xvii
Instructor's Guide xix

Introduction Principles of Adult Learning 1
Module 1 The Process of Normal Aging 7
Module 2 Communicating Effectively 25
Module 3 Understanding and Identifying Depression and Recognizing the Risk of Suicide 37
Module 4 Understanding Alzheimer's Disease and Other Dementias 53
Module 5 Caring for Confused Older Adults 65
Module 6 The Effect of Medication on Older Adults 77
Module 7 Understanding and Recognizing Alcohol Abuse 91
Module 8 Understanding and Recognizing Elder Abuse 103
Module 9 Ethical Issues in Caring for Older Adults 115
Module 10 Dealing with Death and Dying 123
Module 11 Managing Caregiver Stress 131
Training Materials 141
References 233
Suggested Reading 235
Index 243

List of Tables and Figures

Introduction
Table 1 Characteristics and needs of adult education students 2
Figure 1 Preparation tasks for holding an in-service 6

Module 1 The Process of Normal Aging
Figure 2 Facts about older Americans 8
Table 2 Vision changes and ways to help 15
Table 3 Hearing changes and ways to help 18
Table 4 Taste and smell changes and ways to help 19
Table 5 Skin and nail changes and ways to help 20
Table 6 Respiratory changes and ways to help 20
Table 7 Cardiovascular changes and ways to help 21
Table 8 Gastrointestinal changes and ways to help 21
Table 9 Genitourinary changes and ways to help 23
Table 10 Neurological changes and ways to help 23
Table 11 Musculoskeletal changes and ways to help 24

Module 2 Communicating Effectively
Figure 3 The communication process 26
Figure 4 Techniques to improve communication with clients who have hearing loss 31
Figure 5 Barriers to effective communication 32
Figure 6 Effective listening skills 33
Figure 7 Active listening behaviors 34

Module 3 Understanding and Identifying Depression and Recognizing the Risk of Suicide
Figure 8 Signs of depression checklist 39
Figure 9 Observations of a depressed person 41
Figure 10 Subjects to talk about with a depressed person 44
Figure 11 Ways to help a depressed person 47
Figure 12 The warning signs of suicide 48
Figure 13 Model suicide-prevention policy 49
Table 12 "I Know" questions and answers 51

Module 4 Understanding Alzheimer's Disease and Other Dementias
Figure 14 Memory loss symptoms 55
Figure 15 Causes of dementia 56
Figure 16 Segments of the brain 60
Figure 17 The function of nerve cells 61
Table 13 Stages and characteristics of Alzheimer's disease 63

Module 5 Caring for Confused Older Adults
Figure 18 Communication problems of people with dementia 67
Figure 19 Techniques of communicating successfully with people with dementia 67
Figure 20 Causes and triggers of behavior problems in people with dementia 69
Figure 21 Purposes of leisure activities 74
Figure 22 101 ways to use remaining capabilities of people with dementia 75

Module 6 The Effect of Medication on Older Adults
Table 14 Reasons for medication abuse and misuse 80
Figure 23 Sample of a chart used for tracking client medication regimen ... 82
Figure 24 Signs and symptoms of potential medication abuse and misuse 85
Figure 25 Medication abuse and misuse—how to help 88

Module 7 Understanding and Recognizing Alcohol Abuse
Figure 26 Facts about alcoholism 93
Figure 27 Barriers to the treatment of alcohol abuse 94
Figure 28 Characteristics of an older abuser of alcohol 95
Figure 29 Special risk factors of alcoholism and older people 97
Figure 30 Signs of an alcohol problem 98
Figure 31 Some interventions and treatments for alcohol abuse 101

Module 8 Understanding and Recognizing Elder Abuse
Figure 32 Types of elder abuse reported 105
Table 15 Types of abuse, neglect, and exploitation 106
Figure 33 Abuser's relationship to the victim 107
Figure 34 Percentage of abusive women versus abusive men 107
Table 16 Characteristics of the abuser and the victim 108
Figure 35 Percentage of abused women versus abused men 109
Figure 36 Profile of elder abuse victims; types of disability 109
Figure 37 Signs of physical abuse 110
Figure 38 Typical abusive behaviors of family member or caregiver 111
Figure 39 Indicators of financial exploitation 111

Module 9 Ethical Issues in Caring for Older Adults
Figure 40 Myths and facts regarding sexuality and older people 121
Figure 41 Ethical behavior regarding the acceptance of money and gifts by caregivers 122

Module 10 Dealing with Death and Dying
Table 17 Stages of grief 125

Module 11 Managing Caregiver Stress
Figure 42 Diseases that are induced by stress 132
Figure 43 Changes in the human body that are induced by stress 133
Table 18 Signs of stress 134
Figure 44 Ways a caregiver can manage her time more efficiently 136
Figure 45 Relaxation techniques that can be used by professional caregivers to reduce stress 137

List of Activities

Module 1 The Process of Normal Aging

Attitudes Toward Aging 9

Stereotypes of Aging 9

Facts on Aging 10

Module 2 Communicating Effectively

Discussion of Communication Problems 27

Test Your Observation and Reporting Skills 27

Positive Feedback 28

Word Meanings 28

Tearing a Sheet of Paper 29

Ways of Communicating 30

Communication Vignette 31

Active Listening 34

Module 3 Understanding and Identifying Depression and Recognizing the Risk of Suicide

Case Study 42

Focusing on the Client 45

Stress Monitoring 50

"I Know" 50

Module 4 Understanding Alzheimer's Disease and Other Dementias

The Confused Mind—What Is It Like? 62

Module 5 Caring for Confused Older Adults

Guess My Line 66

Role Play 68

Task Analysis 72

Module 6 The Effect of Medication on Older Adults

True or False Quiz 79

Take Your Medicine! 84

Misuse or Not? 86

Effective Communication 89

Module 7 Understanding and Recognizing Alcohol Abuse
Beliefs About Alcohol Problems 92
Use or Abuse 99

Module 8 Understanding and Recognizing Elder Abuse
Is This Elder Abuse? 104
Is This a Risky Situation? 113

Module 9 Ethical Issues in Caring for Older Adults
Origins of Ethics 116
Values Clarification Exercise 117
Confidentiality Case Studies 118
Code of Ethics 119
Sexuality in Older People: A Case Study 121
Acceptance of Gifts: A Case Study 122

Module 10 Dealing with Death and Dying
Reminiscing 124
Responses to Dying 127
Special Needs of Terminally Ill People and Their Families 128

Module 11 Managing Caregiver Stress
Measuring Coping Strategies 135
Self-Care Inventory 135
Tense Situations 139

About the Authors

Ellen Cervantes, M.S.W., is the Supervisor of The Center for Applied Gerontology, a division of the Council for Jewish Elderly, Chicago. She joined the Center in 1990 after serving as the Educator for the Council's Living-at-Home Program, and is responsible for designing and coordinating monthly educational programs for practitioners in the field of gerontology on medical, policy, and counseling issues.

Ms. Cervantes received her master's degree in social work from the University of California, Berkeley, in 1977. After receiving her degree, she was appointed Program Coordinator for the Brotherhood Way Jewish Community Center in San Francisco. She became the Director of the Berkeley Jewish Community Center in 1980. In 1982 Ms. Cervantes moved to Chicago in order to use her group work and education skills at the Board of Jewish Education, the Jewish Family Service, and the Council for Jewish Elderly.

As a volunteer, Ms. Cervantes has been active on the board of directors of Resolve of Illinois, an organization that provides information and support to people with infertility problems.

Ms. Cervantes contributed "The home care paraprofessional and adult learning principles" to *Challenges and innovations in home care,* Beverly Hills, CA: Sage Publications (1994) (with Charlotte Schuerman); "Respite care—What is it and why use it" to *Elder Care Service 1990–1991, The greater Chicago area guide to eldercare,* Phoenix: Oryx Press (1990); and *Classic Residence activities manual,* New York: Classic Residence by Hyatt (1989).

Jeanne Heid-Grubman, L.S.W., is the Education Coordinator at The Center for Applied Gerontology, where she coordinates workshops for home care aides, supervisors, and consumers. She has 17 years' experience in the aging field, in both direct service and administration. As Vice President of United Methodist Homes and Services from 1982 to 1991, she was instrumental in developing a comprehensive community health center for senior adults as well as a teaching nursing home model.

Ms. Heid-Grubman is a licensed social worker and nursing home administrator and a certified assisted housing manager. She earned her master's degree from the School of Social Service Administration at the University of Chicago, with an individual specialty in geriatric program planning and administration.

Charlotte K. Schuerman, L.C.S.W., is the Director of Home and Community Based Service, at the Council for Jewish Elderly, Chicago. In addition to supervising The Center for Applied Gerontology and the Living-at-Home Program, she is responsible for the Adult Day Care, In-Home Personal Services, Home Repair, Senior Companion, and the In-Home Shopping Service programs. Her responsibilities include the development of program ideas, management of staff, fundraising, and collaborative ventures with educational institutions, social agencies, and centers on aging.

Prior to working at the Council for Jewish Elderly, Ms. Schuerman was Project Director at the Edwin F. Mandel Legal Aid Clinic of the University of Chicago Law School, where she was responsible for the design and administration of the project. She trained law students and social work students to provide legal and social work services to poor, minority, and chronically mentally ill clients. Ms. Schuerman holds a master's degree in social service administration from the University of Chicago.

Charlotte Schuerman is the coeditor (with J. Hardy) of *Challenges and innovations in homecare,* San Francisco: American Society on Aging (1994), and the coauthor (with Ellen Cervantes) of "Respite care—What is it and why use it" In *Elder services: The greater Chicago area guide to eldercare,* Phoenix: Oryx Press (1990).

Foreword

People who make the greatest difference in the lives of frail, older individuals are the paraprofessionals, who spend the most time assisting them. Yet these in-home workers and nursing facility aides typically receive the least money, fewest hours of training, and minimal recognition for their work. This book seeks to remedy at least one of these deficiencies by providing a useful and readable educational resource.

Training materials of this kind must be practical without being simplistic, and must organize material in a fashion that invites ready access and interaction with the material. Workers on the front line need answers without a lot of jargon, presented in a manner that does not overload them with unnecessary detail. This book exceeds these expectations through a practical, clear, and streamlined text.

Supervisors will find the book provides them with a basis for training new workers and filling in gaps in knowledge for seasoned caregivers. Frontline staff will want to keep a copy on hand for easy reference when questions arise during the course of their service to older adults. A periodic review of key chapters will invigorate staff meetings and provide a structure for stimulating discussion.

As its greatest strength, this book makes use of the fact that paraprofessionals spend more time with older people than any other long-term care providers. Caregivers are encouraged to employ the privileges that arise through close and consistent contact. In the chapter on depression, for example, the adult learner is instructed in how to recognize which behavioral changes should be reported. The intimate nature of their work affords such powers of observation, yet this is the first text that depicts those powers in an educational context and addresses paraprofessionals with respect for their capacities in this area.

I look forward to using the book myself as a training tool and recommending it to others who provide training to paraprofessionals. A text like this has been needed for a long time. I welcome its appearance and applaud its competence.

Wendy Lustbader, M.S.W.
Author of **Counting on Kindness: The Dilemmas of Dependency**

Preface

As the population grows older and more frail, the need for professional caregivers in home health and long-term care also grows. Caregivers serve older people in many capacities, as companion, personal shopper, chef, and homemaker, in a variety of workplaces, such as continuing care communities, nursing homes, and residences. Although the field has developed in tandem with the advances made in aging, gerontology, and the quality of life of older people, little or no specialized training has been made available to care providers. To compensate, many paraprofessionals have extrapolated experience from a related field or have relied on their caring instincts. However, the advances in the field of aging have made it difficult for care providers to rely solely on instinct or experience for guidance in their work. This book has been written in an attempt to supplement these methods by providing an in-service manual for trainers of care workers in the field of aging.

In developing training materials suitable for the paraprofessional working with older people, the authors have found that experiential education works best for adult learners and have employed the techniques of experiential education in writing this book. This type of education joins what the learner knows from experience to the didactic content of classroom information. The authors designed 11 modules that cover the situations most often faced by care providers in their work, such as dealing with older adults with dementia, alcoholism, and depression; how to better communicate with older people; what a caregiver should do when she observes mental or physical abuse in the home of the older client or when an older person exhibits inappropriate behavior; how to handle a client who is abusing medication; relaxation techniques that the caregiver can use to relieve her own stress; and ways to cope with stressful circumstances or people. Each module contains numerous activities that provide an opportunity to adult learners to cooperate, to role play, to build self-esteem, and to think more deeply about their work, something that is not always available during a busy workday. Trainers also may wish to create activities specific to the interests of their group of adult learners; the list of resources at the back of the book may provide guidance in the development of these activities. An instructor's guide is supplied prior to the Introduction to assist trainers in using this book and setting up in-service sessions.

The authors would like to thank Cynthia Belle, A.C.C.; Maria Betke, R.N., B.S.N.; Michele Bridgeman, B.S.; Sharon Feryance, L.C.S.W.; Lorelei Inda, B.S.; Juliana LaPuma, R.N., M.A.; Sherry Lopata, R.N., B.S.N.; Deborah Sitz,

R.N., M.S.N.; and Georgia Vayette, B.A., for their contributions to this manual. Their dedication to their craft and enjoyment of care providers shines through in their work. Our thanks also go to the women and men who do this sometimes thankless job with wholehearted concern and kindness.

Instructor's Guide

This manual can be used for teaching caregivers in both community-based and residential long-term care facilities. The training modules appear in a recommended training progression; however, they can be used in any order. Each module is designed to be used by itself for a 90-minute-long training session. The teaching goal and objectives for the module are identified on the first page, followed by a glossary of key terms introduced in the module. Experiential activities are integrated into the text. Handout materials ("Training Materials") that are ready for photoduplication can be found at the back of the book, along with resources and further reading for the instructor. Permission from the publisher to use these materials for in-service workshops is not necessary. (You may want to make a master copy of each handout and store the masters in a folder. The handouts also may be used as an overhead projection.)

In order to make the training directly relevant to your group, add discussion time so that concerns and ideas of the learners can be addressed. Experiment with the activities included (marked with a starburst symbol) to bring the points home to your staff while facilitating their integration of new ideas.

Because most older people receiving care and most of their care providers are women, we have chosen to use feminine pronouns in most cases. In community-based care the caregiver may be referred to as the homemaker, home care worker, home care aide, or the home health aide. In a nursing home the caregiver is generally called the nursing assistant or the nursing aide. We have chosen to refer to the person providing care as the "care provider" or "caregiver," a general term that is applicable to any of these job titles.

The Paraprofessional in Home Health and Long-Term Care

Introduction

Principles of Adult Learning

Tell me, and I'll forget. Show me, and I may not remember. Involve me, and I'll understand.

—Native American saying

Continuing in-service education for care providers is a critical issue. In planning an in-service, it is important to pay attention to the established principles of adult learning. Many care providers have not been in a formal school setting for years, and adult education is different from traditional forms of education.

First, some students may resist learning something new. Even if their old way of doing things is not correct or efficient, it is predictable. The person knows what to do and what to expect. Change is unpredictable and therefore frightening.

Second, some adults may lack self-confidence as students. They may have had negative experiences with education in their earlier years. This situation may make them cautious about participating in class discussions and other exercises.

Third, adult learners have many responsibilities and distractions in their lives. Just getting them to attend the in-service in the first place may be a challenge. Once there, they may be very difficult to engage because of their fatigue and stress. (See Table 1 for more details on the learning needs of adult students.)

These challenges notwithstanding, care providers can be eager and appreciative learners. Under the right circumstances, there will be lively and thoughtful discussions, active participation in exercises and group activities, and a willingness to share experiences with one another. The following teaching techniques are effective in developing this kind of classroom environment.

Table 1. Characteristics and needs of adult education students

General characteristics	Basic needs
Declining vision, hearing, reaction time Slower to learn	Creature comforts in classroom. No smoking. Warm-up time. Patient instructor.
Attention span of 15–18 minutes	Freedom and spontaneity in classroom. Breaks.
Individualistic and self-directed	Desire and opportunity to learn new subject. Support and respect for individual in heterogeneous group.
Have own beliefs and customs	Teacher-directed learning about cultural differences: speech, eye contact, body language, time consciousness, etc. Teacher recognizes, accepts, and uses differences to advantage of students.
More experienced in life	Teacher knowledgeable, sincere, and enthusiastic to gain learners' respect.
Can draw from experience and learn from other students	Role playing. Group discussion; learning center in classroom.
Nervous about change and accepting new learning	Sensible goals that satisfy personal needs.
Sense of past failures	Repeated successes, confidence and security, recognition of contributions.
Cautious about speaking in class to avoid failure and to maintain self-esteem	Motivation by acceptance, praise, and respect.
Oriented toward people and problems	Problem-solving approach to address realistic experiences.
Prefer immediate application of learning	Variety of practical, hands-on activities.
Memory by meaningful association	Variety of sensory stimuli, questions and cause and effect. Objects, pictures, and multimedia instructional aids.
Have other responsibilities and distractions	Flexibility and individual attention from teacher. Learner-centered assignments.

Creating an Open and Accepting Atmosphere

The instructor is responsible for creating a safe context in which to explore and discuss issues. He or she sets the proper mood and tone through displaying good listening skills and respect for the worker. Class participation and sharing of thoughts must be encouraged.

Even intense emotions and strong opinions must be met with acceptance. Criticism of a learner's opinions or comments will serve only to discourage future participation. Respect and openness for different opinions and points of view will serve as an example of appropriate communication.

Call Upon the Learners' Life Experiences

Students learn from one another while reinforcing their own self-confidence. They must be able to make a connection between the content presented and their own life experiences. The new knowledge, skills, and attitudes will become part of their lives only if they seem relevant. Hearing others relate stories similar to their own helps learners realize that they are not alone.

Explain the Usefulness of the Material Taught

Adult learners are practical. They want to know why they need to learn something before they will enthusiastically participate in the learning process. Therefore, instructors should explain the objectives of the learning session and encourage participants to make comments and ask questions. The instructor must impress learners with the significance of the information being taught; the students must learn how and when to use the new material.

Use a Variety of Teaching Techniques

To compensate for the shorter average attention spans of adult education students, oral presentation should be supplemented with other delivery methods. Examples include small group discussions, brainstorming sessions, practice drills, and class exercises.

Use Visual Aids to Reinforce What Is Being Said

A common rule of thumb about presentations is that people remember

- 20% of what they hear
- 50% of what they hear and see
- 90% of what they hear, see, and do

Visual aids may take many forms, including the following:

- **Flip chart and blackboard** Audiences can accept information at four or five times the rate at which the average speaker talks. These two types of visual aids increase learning comprehension and retention by involving the mind's excess capacity to learn. Recording comments from the group reinforces key concepts and encourages participants to build new ideas from those written down. Also, flip charts and blackboards are inexpensive and convenient.
- **Overhead projector** Using an overhead projector during a lecture highlights key points and takes advantage of both the auditory and the visual senses. Graphs, diagrams, and cartoons can be displayed on an overhead as additional reinforcement of the material being covered. Participants' ideas are easily recorded on a transparency.
- **Videotape** Video provides an effective way to communicate new ideas or model positive behavior. It saves time by relaying a message quickly, clearly, and succinctly. Video offers an alternate approach to learning, allowing your training to reflect the fact that different people learn in differ-

ent ways: some by reading, some by observing, and some by doing. Video pulls together several approaches to learning. Watching a videotape allows viewers to observe situations that they could not otherwise enter. Coupled with discussion, video produces an engaging learning experience. There are four good times to show a video:

1. To kick off a session
2. To close a session
3. Just before lunch
4. At big meetings

The one bad time to show a video is after lunch. In a dark, quiet room, people who have just eaten are likely to fall asleep.

- **Handouts** An outline of the lecture material, with sufficient space for note taking, enhances the participant's ability to learn relatively difficult material. Handouts can also summarize content, emphasize a point, or provide supplemental information. Adult learners like to take something "concrete" away from the class.

Offer Opportunities to Experience or Practice What Is Being Taught

The best way to explain new ideas and to reinforce previously introduced verbal or visual concepts is to include an experiential exercise. This approach brings concepts to life and allows participants to hone new skills and discuss and integrate new ideas. Each module in this text includes experiential exercises. Use the exercises that best fit your group. Feel free to experiment—add your own exercises and modify exercises so that they relate to the concerns or needs of your students. Allow adequate time to talk about feelings, thoughts, and actions generated by the experiential exercises.

Suggested exercises include the following:

- **Practice sessions** Have participants practice the skills and techniques they have learned.
- **Role playing** Participants assume the parts of various characters. They then enact the scenes based on their experience or on what they consider to be the correct approach. Assign other people in the room to comment on the role playing. Ask for suggestions of alternative ways to handle the situation. People who make suggestions can be asked to act them out.
- **Small group discussion** Have small groups answer a series of questions to focus on key elements or ideas. Have each small group appoint a spokesperson to report to the entire group.

TEACHING TIPS

Be prepared to limit self-disclosure. When self-disclosure seems too personal and too private, feel free to interrupt the person's story with an empathic response. Use the person's comment to emphasize a teaching point that is appropriate to the content of what has been shared. This approach will redirect the discussion back to the larger group and help you return to your structured teaching plan.

Also, be ready to deal with learners who monopolize the discussion. A monopolizer gives you an opportunity to model respect for different opinions and viewpoints. Use the same method outlined for excessive self-disclosure to handle a monopolizer. If the monopolizer cannot be redirected, interrupt again with an apology, such as "What you are sharing is important, and I'm sorry that we do not have more time to hear about your experience. Unfortunately, I need to move on" or "Maybe we could talk more about this during the break or after class." At this point, use body language to reinforce your need to move on. Stop making eye contact, turn your body slightly away from the person, and direct your conversation to the larger group.

The physical comfort of the learning environment (including appropriate temperature, lighting, ventilation, and seating arrangements) enhances learning. If possible, participants should not be seated in strict columns and rows. Arrange chairs and tables in a circle or square, with chairs on the outside facing in whenever possible. Providing a variety of activities and taking regular breaks also improves the learning atmosphere.

Participant body language will show interest or fatigue. A good instructor will be aware of these signals and will adapt presentation style and methods to encourage learning and participation. For a longer in-service, a break should be offered when the participants begin showing signs of restlessness.

Thorough preparation is essential to an effective in-service. If overlooked, seemingly small details can cause major problems in the learning environment. See Figure 1 for a list of tasks that must be completed prior to the in-service.

Care providers are a vital part of the health care team. Quality in-service education is a way of enhancing their knowledge and expertise. This way, care providers will be more able to meet the growing needs of clients who choose to stay in their own homes in spite of physical changes that reduce their independence.

- ☐ Prepare a flyer announcing the in-service.
- ☐ Arrange for flyer to be given to each participant at least 2 weeks in advance.
- ☐ Determine whether an overhead projector and screen are available.
  - If so, prepare overhead transparencies from masters in back of book.
  - If not, make arrangements for displaying material on flip chart or blackboard.
- ☐ Order refreshments, if applicable.
- ☐ Visit the workshop site and check for availability or location of the following:
  - Seating arrangements
  - Electrical outlets
  - Projector stand or table
  - Easel for flip chart
  - Space for unit activities
  - Thermostat
  - Light switches
  - Table or podium for speaker
- ☐ Copy handouts for distribution.
- ☐ Arrange room and equipment.
- ☐ Prepare registration material.

Figure 1. Preparation tasks for holding an in-service.

Module 1

The Process of Normal Aging

Goal:

To review commonly held impressions about older people and to develop empathy for their special needs

Objectives:

1. To identify common misconceptions about aging
2. To state the facts about aging and older people
3. To understand certain deficits commonly experienced by older adults

Key Terms

Ageism: Making assumptions about an older person.
Empathy: Understanding and being sensitive to the feelings, thoughts, and experiences of another person.
Osteoporosis: A condition that is characterized by decreased bone mass and decreased bone density, causing bones to become fragile.
Stereotype: Commonly held assumption that is not necessarily based on fact.

As older adults become an ever-larger part of the American population, the need to understand older people and their special problems also increases. Figure 2 contains a list of facts about older adults, derived from the National Center for Health Statistics.

STEREOTYPES ABOUT OLDER ADULTS

Most of us make judgments about people based on our beliefs. We may not even be aware that we are doing this. Care providers who see frail, depressed, or belligerent older people nearly every day may come to believe that they are seeing a picture of normal aging. This negative image can inhibit a worker from approaching each new client with an open mind and can prevent her

- In 1992 there were more than 30 million persons over 65. By the year 2000, there will be more than 34 million.
- One out of every eight persons is 65 years of age or older.
- About 5%, or a little over 1 million, of people over 65 years old live in institutions of one kind or another.
- About 9 million older persons live alone or with nonrelatives.
- There are 150 older women for every 100 older men.
- Most older men are married. Most older women are widowed. Also, there are five times as many widows as widowers, and half of all women in this group are widows.
- Of all older adults, 86% suffer from one or more chronic health conditions of varying degrees of severity.
- Of all people over 65 years old, 23% are limited in their activities of daily living due to chronic health conditions.
- Of all people over age 85, 49% have difficulty with the activities of daily living.
- Among people over 65, 41% of the women live alone, as compared to 16% of the men.
- The majority of people over age 65 who live alone will eventually be institutionalized.
- The fastest-growing age group of the population of the United States is adults over 85 years.
- In 1980 over 2.5 million people, or 10% of the population 65 and older, were nonwhite. It is expected that by 2050, 15% will be nonwhite, and by 2050, 20%.
- People over 65 go to doctors an average of eight times a year, compared to five times a year for people under 65.
- People over 65 are hospitalized twice as often as people under 65, their hospital visits average 50% longer, and they use twice as many prescription drugs.

Figure 2. Facts about older Americans. (Adapted from National Center for Health Statistics.)

from being able to focus on the strengths of each person. Talking about one's attitudes toward aging enables a person to go beyond preconceived notions of aging to see each individual as he or she is. The Attitudes Toward Aging activity can help you get a sense of any stereotypes that your in-service learners may have. Allow 10 to 15 minutes for participants to respond to the questions in the handout. Then discuss responses.

ATTITUDES TOWARD AGING

- Distribute handout "Attitudes Toward Aging."
- Allow 10–15 minutes for students to answer questions.
- Conduct a discussion based on the handout.

1. What makes a person seem young?
2. What makes a person seem old?
3. Think about two people you know who are in their 70s. One seems young, and one seems old. Why?
4. What do older people have now that they did not have when they were younger?
5. What did older people have when they were younger that they do not have now?
6. Imagine yourself as an older person. What will you do for enjoyment? With whom will you spend your time? Where will you live?
7. What do you fear most about aging?
8. What do you look forward to in your older years?
9. How do your attitudes about aging affect your work with older people?

Along with our own perceptions, we must deal with the negative stereotypes of aging that our society presents. A stereotype is a widely accepted notion that is not necessarily based in fact.

We make assumptions about people based upon their age. Many people think that older adults are all alike. In fact, people begin to differ more from each other as they age, rather than becoming more alike. Making assumptions about an older person is called *ageism*. Most of us, even those of us who work with older adults, are guilty of some degree of ageism.

STEREOTYPES OF AGING

- Have the group brainstorm stereotypes of aging. List participants' responses on a flip chart or the blackboard.
- Show several examples of birthday cards that show negative stereotypes of aging.
- Discuss some vibrant, intelligent older people of today and the past. Some examples are Paul Newman, movie star, champion racing car driver, and food manufacturer; George Burns, come-

dian, who won an Academy Award at age 82; Lee Iacocca, former president of Chrysler Corporation; Ella Fitzgerald, pop/jazz singer; Bob Hope, comedian; and former President George Bush. Ask for additional examples from the group.

Attitudes toward older adults may be based on previous experience, what is seen on television and in movies, and cultural stereotypes. These attitudes may also be based on myths. However, factual information can counteract the stereotypes about aging.

FACTS ON AGING

- Pass out copies of the handout "What's Your Aging I.Q.?"
- Give participants 15–20 minutes to complete the quiz.
- Discuss questions and answers with the learners.

1. Baby boomers are the fastest-growing segment of the population.

   False. There are more than 3 million Americans over the age of 85. That number is expected to quadruple by the year 2040, when there will be more than 12 million people in that age group. People age 85 and older are the fastest-growing age group in the United States.

2. Families do not bother with their older relatives.

   False. Most people live close to their parents and see them often. Many older adults live with their spouses. An estimated 80% of men and 60% of women live in family settings. Only 5% of the older population live in nursing homes.

3. All people become confused or forgetful if they live long enough.

   False. Confusion and serious forgetfulness in old age may result from Alzheimer's disease or other conditions that cause irreversible damage to the brain. At least 100 other problems can bring on the same symptoms—for example, minor head injuries, high fever, poor nutrition, adverse drug reactions, and depression. These conditions are treatable, however, and the confusion they cause can be eliminated.

4. A person can be too old to exercise.

   False. Exercise at any age can help strengthen the heart and lungs and lower blood pressure. Exercises can also improve muscle strength and, if carefully chosen, decrease bone loss.

5. Heart disease is a much bigger problem for older men than for older women.

False. The risk of heart disease increases dramatically for women after menopause. By age 65, both men and women have a one-in-three chance of showing symptoms. Maintaining a healthy diet and exercising can significantly reduce the risk of heart disease.

6. The older you get, the less you sleep.

   False. In later life, it is the quality of sleep that declines, not total sleep time. Researchers have found that sleep becomes more fragmented as people age. Many reports suggest that older people are less likely than younger people to stay awake throughout the day; older people also tend to take more naps than younger people do.

7. People should watch their weight as they age.

   True. Most people gain weight as they age. Because of changes in the body and decreasing physical activity, older people usually need fewer calories. Still, a balanced diet is important. Older people require essential nutrients just as younger adults do. An older adult should be concerned about his or her weight if there has been an involuntary gain or loss of 10 pounds or more in the past 6 months.

8. Most older people are depressed. Why not?

   False. Most older people are not depressed. When depression does occur, it is treatable throughout the life cycle by using a variety of approaches, such as family support, psychotherapy, or antidepressant medications. A physician can decide whether a prescribed medication, physical illness, stress, or other factors are causing the depression.

9. There is no point in screening older people for cancer because they cannot be treated.

   False. Many older people can beat cancer, especially if it is found early. Over half of all cancers occur in people 65 and older, which means that screening for cancer in this age group is especially important.

10. Older people take more medications than younger people do.

    True. Older people often have a combination of conditions that require drugs. They consume 25% of all medications and can have many problems with adverse reactions.

11. People begin to lose interest in sex around age 55.

    False. Most older people can—and want to—lead an active, satisfying sex life.

12. If your parents had Alzheimer's disease, you will inevitably get it.

    False. The majority of people with Alzheimer's disease did not inherit the disorder. Scientists have seen an extremely high incidence of the disease in a few families and have identified genes in these families that they think may be responsible.

13. Diet and exercise reduce the risk of osteoporosis.

    True. Women are particularly vulnerable to osteoporosis. They can help prevent bone loss by eating foods rich in calcium and exercising regularly throughout life. Foods such as milk and other dairy products, dark green leafy vegetables, salmon, sardines, and tofu promote new bone growth. Activities such as walking, biking, and simple exercises to strengthen the upper body can also be effective.

14. As your body changes with age, so does your personality.

    False. Research has found that, except for the changes that can result from Alzheimer's disease and other similar conditions, personality is one of the few constants of life.

15. Older people might as well accept urinary accidents as a fact of life.

    False. Urinary incontinence is a symptom, not a disease. Usually it is caused by specific changes in body function that can result from infection, diseases, pregnancy, or the use of certain medications. A variety of treatment options is available for people who seek medical attention.

16. Suicide is mainly a problem for teenagers.

    False. Suicide is most prevalent among people age 65 and older. An older person's concern with suicide should be taken very seriously, and professional help should be sought quickly.

17. Falls and injuries "just happen" to older people.

    False. Falls are the most common cause of injuries for people over age 65. However, many of these injuries, which often include broken bones, are avoidable. Good safety habits and regular vision and hearing tests can help prevent accidents. Knowing whether medications affect balance and coordination is also a good idea.

18. Everybody gets cataracts.

    False. Not everyone gets cataracts, although many older people do. Some 18% of people between the ages of 65 and 74 have cataracts, while more than 40% of those between 75 and

85 have this problem. Surgery is an effective treatment for cataracts; more than 90% of people who undergo the operation say they can see better after this corrective procedure.

19. Extremes of heat and cold can be especially dangerous for older people.

    True. The body's thermostat functions less efficiently with age, making the older person's body less able to adapt to heat or cold.

20. "You can't teach an old dog new tricks."

    False. People at any age can learn new information and skills. Research suggests that older people can build new skills and improve old ones, including how to use a computer.

EMPATHY

Empathy is the ability to relate to another person's emotions, thoughts, and feelings. Empathy is different from sympathy, which implies feeling sorry for a person. Although the difference is subtle, it is important. Along with empathy comes understanding. If a caregiver understands what it is like to struggle with physical and mental impairments, she will have more patience with her clients. It is helpful to imagine experiencing the same problems. This is the notion of "walking in their shoes."

The Sensory Dysfunction Exercise activity is designed to give participants a taste of what it feels like to do daily activities while dealing with vision loss or paralysis. These are two types of disabilities common to older people (Richman & Glantz, 1992b). Caregivers are surprised by the amount of energy it takes to complete simple tasks, such as getting dressed, when afflicted by a partial paralysis. They often comment on the discomfort of feeling so dependent upon the people who are helping them around. For the participants, these losses are only temporary. However, they do bring up many of the feelings experienced by older people needing care. The materials needed for this exercise include the following:

- Pair of used eyeglasses
- Petroleum jelly
- Yarn balls
- Comb
- Roll of adhesive tape
- Lipstick
- Fingernail file
- Oversized shirt to go over clothing
- Safety pins
- Juice bottle
- Wheelchair

Pass out copies of the Activity handout, and have learners follow the directions indicated in the handout and listed here (Richman & Glantz, 1992b).

Blindfolded and with guidance of a partner:

1. Go to washroom and use it.
2. Walk around room, through narrow space, through a doorway.
3. Ascend and descend stairs.
4. Walk to table and chairs, sit down.
5. Cut five pieces of yarn measured between tape.

With right arm and leg totally "paralyzed," sitting in a wheelchair:

1. Put on and remove a shirt, buttoning and unbuttoning the buttons.
2. File your nails.
3. Wheel your wheelchair 10 feet: forward, backward, right, and left.

First with smeared glasses and gloves, then with taped fingers:

1. Go to your purse or pocket, take out four coins, and identify them.
2. Open and close a safety pin and a bottle.
3. Button and unbutton four buttons on the shirt.

With blocked visual-field glasses:

1. Comb your hair or put on lipstick.
2. Write your name.

Afterwards, ask participants what they learned about the problem of completing "simple" tasks while struggling with a partial disability.

Even with some degree of disability, a person has remaining strengths and capabilities. The role of the care provider is to make use of the skills and strengths of the older person. A worker can discuss these with the client and suggest adaptations to the client's environment that will enhance his or her independence. Empathy and knowledge help a worker to "do with" a client, rather than always "do for."

The care provider who understands the normal physical changes associated with aging can identify the signs of abnormal changes. She will be better able to notice when there is a problem and then can report it to a supervisor or family member.

Rehabilitation Associates has developed an extensive series of charts on sensory deficits that can occur as people age and ways caregivers can help. The charts discuss the normal changes of aging and the sensory deficits common to an aging body (see Tables 2–11 at the end of the module). Also suggested are ways to enhance the remaining capabilities of the older person. The areas of capability covered are visual, auditory, taste and smell, skin and nails, respiratory, cardiovascular, gastrointestinal, genitourinary, neurological, and musculoskeletal (Richman & Glantz, 1992a).

In this module the care provider has been asked to look at the stereotypes about aging that she might hold. Learners have been asked to discuss their fears about their own aging and have had a review of the normal physical changes associated with the aging body. All these exercises and information sheets can enable the caregiver to see beyond the stereotype to the person inside the body. With an empathic attitude, the care provider will be better able to personalize the care given and enhance the capabilities of the person receiving care.

Table 2. Vision changes and ways to help

Vision changes	Ways to help
• As a person ages, the lens in the eye yellows and thickens. The muscles that control pupil size also weaken. As a result, the older eye requires more light than the young eye. To see clearly, a 65-year-old eye needs more than twice as much light as a 20-year-old eye.	• Provide adequate lighting. Be aware of poor lighting and that the older person may be unable to see obstacles, read signs, or recognize familiar people when the lighting is poor.
• The lens grows unevenly and becomes striated. The lens tends to refract the light that passes through it, causing glare problems. A small amount of glare that may hardly bother a younger person may cause great difficulties for the older person. Glare also may cause anxiety and inability to concentrate.	• Carefully adjust shades or drapes throughout the day to avoid glare from windows. Avoid shiny surfaces that reflect light. Tabletops, waxed floors, vinyl upholstery, and mirrors may create glare. • Sunglasses, big-brimmed hats, or sunshades may help when clients are outdoors or riding in a car. When clients cannot express themselves, caregivers must watch for signs of anxiety due to glare.
• Changes in the lens make color perception more difficult. Pastel colors (pink, yellow, pale blue) may all look alike. Brown, dark blue, and black may be difficult to identify correctly.	• Do not interpret inability to identify colors as a sign of confusion. • Do not expect older people to use pastels and very dark colors in a color-coding system. Clients should not depend upon color to help them take the correct pill.
• The older eye does not adapt quickly to changes in light levels. Abrupt changes can be hazardous and may cause falls and other accidents.	• Place lights strategically and keep some lights on so that changes in lighting will be more gradual. For example, nightlights in bedrooms will help. • When there is an abrupt change in the light level, an older person should wait until the eyes have adapted before continuing to walk. • Be careful when placing furniture just inside an entryway. An older person who enters a building may bump into things that are just inside the door if his or her eyes have not yet adjusted to the change in lighting.
• Conditions of the eye that cause vision loss are very common among older people. However, most older	• Older people should have their eyes examined by an ophthalmologist regularly. *(continued)*

Table 2. *continued*

Vision changes	Ways to help
people are not totally blind and can be taught to use their residual vision. Over half of the severe visual impairments occur in people 65 and over. Legal blindness is most common in this age group. The changes in vision occur slowly, and older people are often unaware of them.	• Moving closer to things is one of the best ways to see them better. • Extra-large things are easier to see. These include large-print dials, controls, and buttons. • Contrasting colors make things easier to see. For example, doorways can contrast with the wall, wall sides can contrast with the tablecloth, the chair seat can contrast with the floor, and personal items can contrast with a covering on the dresser top. • Avoid clutter. It is difficult to distinguish crowded items. • Don't change the furniture arrangement unless it is necessary; if you do, ensure that older people become familiar with the new layout.
• Glaucoma is an insidious eye disease that has no noticeable symptoms until irreversible damage is done. It involves a loss of vision due to raised intraocular pressure, which damages the optic nerve. Glaucoma can be controlled and vision loss prevented if it is detected in time.	• There is currently a simple and painless test for glaucoma that older adults should be made aware of. They should also realize the importance of having the test.
• At this time there is no known prevention for cataracts, but they can be successfully treated by the surgical removal of the lens that has become cloudy and opaque. The surgery is usually performed when the vision loss has become severe. The lack of a natural lens in the eye is compensated for by special optical lenses that can be recognized by their thickness and the magnification of the person's eyes behind them.	• If a person has had cataract surgery and wears the special glasses, he or she may still experience some difficulty seeing. The person may need help reading, crossing the street, and doing other things that we assume should be easy. Those wearing the special lenses may also be unsure of themselves and want extra reassurance or assistance. However, people who are very proud may need extra assistance but may refuse to ask for it. Ask people how they might be assisted.
• Cataract glasses make objects seem larger. It is sometimes difficult for an older person to adjust to these distortions. A person wearing cataract glasses also has a blind spot at each side where the glasses cannot provide correction. This situation causes things to appear suddenly—to pop into a person's visual field. There is a new technique of implanting a lens in the eye at the time of surgery that has proven very successful. With implanted lenses, some of the problems of visual field change and size distortions are solved.	• Some people are self-conscious about the fact that the lenses make their eyes appear large and may need reassurance. • To avoid startling someone who wears cataract glasses, approach slowly from the front, rather than from the side.

(*continued*)

Table 2. *continued*

Vision changes	Ways to help
• Macular degeneration is a condition that causes loss of central vision as the macula, the area of the retina responsible for central vision, deteriorates. This condition is neither preventable nor curable. It will not, however, cause total blindness because peripheral vision is not affected. A current method being tested to slow the advance of macular degeneration uses a laser to cauterize the hemorrhaging blood vessels in the retina.	• It may be reassuring to tell the person that he or she will not be totally blind from the disease but will retain peripheral vision. • Low-vision aids such as magnifying glasses can be of some help to those in the less-advanced stages of macular degeneration. • Persons with macular degeneration may seem not to have a severe vision problem. Due to their peripheral vision, they can move around independently without bumping into things and may appear to see quite well. When they talk about their vision problems, other people may not believe them and think they are looking for unnecessary extra help or attention.
• There is some indication that a relationship exists between visual loss and mental function.	• Compensation and correction for vision problems may possibly lead to better mental functioning. It is worth a try.
• Persons who have visual deficits are unable to benefit from the nonverbal feedback important to communication. They cannot see the smiles, frowns, or other facial expressions that are an important part of conversation.	• When conversing with persons who have vision problems, use touch to compensate. For example, holding, squeezing, or patting someone's hand lets the person know where you are and assures the person that you have not walked away.
• Dining can present special problems for people with visual impairments. These people may have difficulty eating independently or be afraid to dine socially because they might spill or make mistakes. Food that is difficult to see is not appealing.	• For those with low vision, place settings should be uncluttered, colors should contrast, and glare should be limited. A tablecloth or place mat can lessen glare. Someone should name the foods and tell where each is located. Finger foods and snack time should be provided regularly to allow people to feel more comfortable about their ability to eat appropriately.
• Those who have vision problems may be unsure of themselves in social situations and may even be fearful if they are in unfamiliar surroundings and situations.	• Help people with vision problems to look attractive, and reassure them honestly about their appearance. Always explain the layout of a room and describe the people who are present and those who will accompany them to social activities. Do not leave them alone until they have someone they can talk with or until they are touching a table, chair, or wall that will help with their orientation.

Adapted from Richman & Glantz, 1992a.

Table 3. Hearing changes and ways to help

Hearing changes	Ways to help
• There is a decline in auditory acuity with age called presbycusis. This age-related hearing loss is usually greater for men than for women. The reason for this decline is not known, but it is suspected that men are exposed to more damaging noise during their lifetimes, possibly resulting from being in the military service or due to the nature of their jobs.	• Any older person may need your help in compensating for hearing loss. While people with visual impairments can compensate by bringing things closer, those with hearing loss cannot similarly compensate. • Speak slowly and clearly, and do not change the topic abruptly. Be sure to face the person at eye level and have light on your face so lipreading is possible. Ask the person what you can do to make hearing easier.
• Hearing loss is worse at high frequencies, meaning that some sounds are heard while others are not. Sounds may be distorted, or heard incorrectly, and thus misinterpreted.	• Try to lower your voice rather than allowing your voice to become high or shrill. Women should be especially careful about this. • A sound system used for music, entertainment, or oral presentations should be adjusted so that the bass and lower tones are predominant.
• People with normal hearing have a wide range between the quietest sound they hear and the loudest, which is painful or irritating. For people with hearing loss, this range may be much narrower. Sounds may have to be quite loud to be heard, and sensitivity is increased. If sounds are even a little louder, they may be too loud to be understood or may even be painful.	• Talk to those people with hearing impairments to find out the optimum tone to use. Do not assume that simply making things louder will solve the problem. • Be aware of the fact that noise or music may be irritating and may cause anxiety for persons with hearing loss, even if it has no effect on you. Be especially aware of this situation when you are working with people who are unable to communicate their needs to you. Note signs of anxiety, and try changing noise levels.
• Hearing loss is greater for consonants than for vowels. *S, Z, T, F,* and *G* sounds are particularly difficult to discriminate, which causes difficulty in hearing words correctly. Words that are similar can be particularly difficult to discriminate.	• People should be aware of the fact that even if sounds can be heard, they may not always be heard correctly. The suggestions previously mentioned can be followed; in addition, it is helpful to limit the competing stimuli of background noise. Choose a quiet, private place for talking.
• Some hearing deficits can be helped by the use of hearing aids, but these must be worn and adjusted correctly in order to help. They also regularly require new batteries. Some people never learn to use their hearing aids correctly, or they do not get new batteries often enough.	• Older persons can purchase hearing aids from reputable firms and should learn their proper use. Family members or caregivers serving older persons should also learn how to help adjust or insert the aid or how to change batteries when it is necessary.
• Some hearing deficits cannot be helped by hearing aids, and the per-	• Encourage the use of nonverbal communication such as big smiles,

(*continued*)

Table 3. *continued*

Hearing changes	Ways to help
son's hearing is so poor that verbal communication is difficult.	waving, pointing, or demonstrating. Offer opportunities for activity and social interaction that require no spoken communication. For example, cooking and cleaning up can be done in complete silence by two or more people who have good understanding and cooperation. Also, use writing as a form of communication. Those who appear to be very impaired can understand written statements and questions.
• Hearing and following a conversation can take tremendous amounts of effort and energy for someone with hearing loss. Motivation, the context of the environment, and general feelings of well-being and energy can make a difference in the ability to understand verbal communication. Lack of any or all of these may result in apparent "selective hearing."	• We should try to be more tolerant of "selective hearing." This syndrome is often annoying for those who interact with people with hearing loss, but in some cases there may be some legitimate reasons for it to occur. • Provide opportunities for people to participate in activities that are enjoyable but require little conversation—for example, playing cards, doing puzzles, preparing food, and taking walks.
• Depression and paranoid reactions are common among older persons with hearing loss. When they cannot hear what is being said, they may begin to think that people are talking about them and saying negative things.	• Do everything possible to compensate hearing loss and to ensure that people know what is going on and what the conversation is about. If the conversation does not concern them, tell them what the topic is so that they will not feel left out or talked about.
• Hearing is important to more than communication. It is a way of getting signals from the environment, so it also relates to safety.	• People who work or live with a person with hearing loss should keep this in mind. People in the community should also realize that when an older person crosses the street, he or she may not hear a car horn.

Adapted from Richman & Glantz, 1992a.

Table 4. Taste and smell changes and ways to help

Taste and smell changes	Ways to help
• There is an indication that the senses of taste and smell decline significantly with age. Older people do not perform as well as young people on tasks involving the identification of odors and tastes of food. The seasoning and foods most often identified by taste and smell were salt (89%), coffee (71%), tomatoes	• Older people probably rely on the appearance of the food for identification and motivation to eat. For people with poor vision, foods may have little or no appeal. • Distinctive textures and temperatures can be important for the identification and enjoyment of food. Ice cream and popcorn are two popular items.

(*continued*)

Table 4. *continued*

Taste and smell changes	Ways to help
(69%), and sugar (57%) (Schiffman, 1989).	
• Poor nutrition can have serious consequences for older people, so it is important that they eat properly. Tasteless foods make eating less enjoyable. Bland, low-salt, and other diet restrictions can also contribute to the undesirability of food.	• A pleasant mealtime atmosphere can make people feel more like eating. Talking about the food, the good taste and smell, can make the food appear to taste better. Condiments and foods with strong flavors may also help to maintain interest in food and eating.
• Poor sense of smell and taste may make it difficult to recognize spoiled foods or odors such as gas. This is a potential hazard for the person who lives alone.	• Older people living alone should be encouraged to be aware of these dangers. They can keep track of the age of food in their refrigerators and check the pilot light of gas stoves regularly. • Families and friends can also help check for odors or spoiled foods whenever they visit.

Adapted from Richman & Glanz, 1992a.

Table 5. Skin and nail changes and ways to help

Skin and nail changes	Ways to help
• As people age, skin loses elasticity, and it becomes thinner and more fragile. The blood flow to the skin decreases. Flat brown spots, often called "age" or "liver spots," appear on the hands and face. Oil production is decreased. The skin tends to become dry and wrinkled, and it looks paler.	• Tissue breakdown and decubitus ulcers can be prevented by ensuring that the older individual has an adequate diet high in protein, carbohydrates, and vitamins. • People who are immobilized need to be turned every 2 hours. Bony prominences should be massaged several times a day to stimulate circulation to pressure areas.
• Sweat glands decrease, and there is an increased risk for heatstroke.	• The older individual should be encouraged to wear a hat when in the sun; to wear light, cool clothing; and to drink sufficient amounts of fluid.
• Nails become thicker, rigid, and more brittle.	• Special care should be given to toenails. They should be soaked in warm water before they are clipped. • Diabetics should have their toenails clipped by a podiatrist.

Adapted from Richman & Glantz, 1992a.

Table 6. Respiratory changes and ways to help

Respiratory changes	Ways to help
• Deep breathing becomes difficult due to skeletal muscles becoming more	• Exercise helps increase the rate and depth of breathing.

(*continued*)

Table 6. *continued*

Respiratory changes	Ways to help
rigid. The chest becomes more rounded in shape. The cough mechanism is less effective due to anatomic and muscle changes.	• Good posture can improve use of lung space. Walking can improve posture.
• As a person ages, there is a decreased pulmonary elasticity. This can be as much as a 50% decrease in functional capacity, resulting in shortness of breath during exertion. There is also a 30% decrease in respiratory fluids, which increases the person's risk for infection. Due to changes in the chest wall, breathing tends to occur more in the upper part of the chest.	• Humidification helps keep the respiratory tract moist so that mucous membranes remain intact and resistant to microbial invasion. • Adequate fluid intake, at least a quart of fluid daily, helps keep mucous membranes hydrated. • When there are upper respiratory secretions, drinking fluids can help thin the secretions for easier expectoration.

Adapted from Richman & Glantz, 1992a.

Table 7. Cardiovascular changes and ways to help

Cardiovascular changes	Ways to help
• There is decreased cardiac output, and the heart pumps with less force. However, heart size does not change. The resting heart rate remains unchanged. More time is required for the heart to return to normal after exertion. The heart valves and blood vessels may become thick and rigid. Systolic blood pressure and diastolic pressure rise, but not excessively. Hypertension is not a part of normal aging. An older individual is considered hypertensive if the blood pressure is 160/90 or above. Decreased arteriole elasticity results in increased peripheral resistance, which is responsible for the normal increase in blood pressure seen in older people.	• Exercise can help prevent heart disease and other vascular diseases. A regular program of vigorous physical activity can raise the blood levels of protective, or "good," HDL cholesterol. • HDL cholesterol can also be raised by lowering body fat and by quitting smoking. • An exercise program can help regulate blood pressure. One study has shown that people who maintain their fitness have a 34% lower risk of developing hypertension. • Older people should not begin a vigorous training program until they have had a medical examination to rule out any conditions that would limit their activity, such as heart disease, and to learn exactly how intense their workouts should be.

Adapted from Richman & Glantz, 1992a.

Table 8. Gastrointestinal changes and ways to help

Gastrointestinal changes	Ways to help
• Tooth enamel thins, and teeth become brittle. However, tooth loss is not a normal aging change.	• Encourage regular dental checkups. Good oral hygiene, including brushing and flossing daily to remove plaque, can prevent tooth decay and gum disease.

(*continued*)

Table 8. *continued*

Gastrointestinal changes	Ways to help
	• Fluoride in drinking water as well as the use of fluoride toothpaste and mouth rinses can prevent tooth decay. • Older individuals with arthritis who find it difficult to hold a toothbrush can be helped by attachments that connect the brush handle to the hand or by enlarging the handle by attaching it to a sponge, styrofoam ball, or similar object. Individuals with limited shoulder movements often find it helpful to lengthen the toothbrush handle by attaching a piece of wood or plastic. Also, electric toothbrushes may be easier to use.
• Saliva production decreases, which can result in dry mouth and decreased taste. Biting force decreases. Gag reflex decreases.	• Seniors who experience dry mouth should consult their doctor or dentist. This problem can be a side effect of many medications and certain medical treatments. Dry mouth can also be helped by drinking extra water and by avoiding sugary snacks, beverages with caffeine, tobacco, and alcohol.
• Changes in the nerves and muscles of the esophagus cause slower swallowing. The area at the bottom of the esophagus may not close properly, allowing food and acid from the stomach to back up into the esophagus, causing heartburn or chest pain. Blood flow to the stomach decreases, and fewer digestive juices are produced. Food remains in the stomach longer. The ability to absorb carbohydrates, fats, vitamin D, and calcium decreases.	• Allow extra time for eating. Sometimes, several small meals during the day are better than three large meals. • Heartburn can be helped by avoiding tomato products, chocolate, fried foods, and peppermint and by stopping smoking. Antacids and sleeping with the head of the bed raised six inches can also help. • Older people should eat slowly and, when possible, try to relax for 30 minutes after each meal.
• The muscle movements of the large bowel slow down (peristalsis), often resulting in constipation. Diverticulosis (small sacs forming on the wall of the large intestine) is a common problem in older people. In diverticulitis, the sacs become inflamed.	• "Regularity" does not mean a daily bowel movement. Normal bowel movement can be as often as three times a day or as little as once a week. • Regularity can be improved by increasing the fluid intake, eating foods high in fiber, and staying physically active.
• Peristalsis, diverticulitis	• Older people should be careful not to misuse laxatives. Self-medication can lead to constipation. • A diet high in fiber with increased fluids is important in the treatment of diverticulosis.

(*continued*)

Table 8. *continued*

Gastrointestinal changes	Ways to help
	• Remember that severe stomach pain is not normal and should be reported to a doctor or nurse.

Adapted from Richman & Glantz, 1992a.

Table 9. Genitourinary changes and ways to help

Genitourinary changes	Ways to help
• As a person ages, the kidneys and bladder become smaller. Therefore, urination can become more frequent. The bladder may not empty completely after voiding, which can result in a urinary tract infection. Weak bladder muscles or other anatomic changes can lead to incontinence.	• Urinary output is affected by kidney function and the amount of fluid intake. Fluid intake should be one and a half quarts or more each day. Older individuals prone to bladder infections should be encouraged to drink cranberry or apple juice, which acidify the urine and discourage bacterial growth. • Incontinence is not an eventuality of aging, though it affects 15–30% of the older population. In many cases incontinence can be cured or at least treated to minimize its detrimental effects. A toileting schedule can be set up to retrain the bladder. • Kegel exercises for women can strengthen the pelvic muscles and help prevent incontinence.
• The prostate enlarges in men as they age and can cause voiding problems. Prostate enlargement is caused by hormonal changes associated with aging. When the problem becomes severe, it can cause bladder outlet obstruction. An enlarged prostate should be screened for cancer by a physician.	• When the problem is not severe, the following interventions can help: (1) Increase fluid intake to prevent infection. (2) Limit drinks containing caffeine, which can cause bladder irritation. (3) Urinate every 2–4 hours to prevent the bladder becoming overdistended. • When prostate enlargement is severe, surgery is the preferred method of alleviating symptoms.

Adapted from Richman & Glantz, 1992a.

Table 10. Neurological changes and ways to help

Neurological changes	Ways to help
• There is a 7% decrease in the size of the brain as we age, and blood flow to the brain may be decreased. Nerve cells are lost. About 10% of	• Recent research on aging has shown that mental sharpness in absence of disease has less to do with aging and more to do with mental inactivity.

(continued)

Table 10. *continued*

Neurological changes	Ways to help
the brain's neurons die every decade of life after 10 years of age. The speed of messages traveling to and from the brain decreases from 10% to 20% over the years. However, studies show that older people perform very well on tests of meaningful memory. It may take them longer to process information, but their ability to learn and retain is as good as that of younger individuals. Excessive loss of memory can result from Alzheimer's disease, other neurological diseases, and acute medical conditions.	• Neurons can grow new connections when stimulated. It is the neuron connections and not the nerve cells themselves that determine how well we think and remember. • The more the brain is challenged, the more it can increase its number of connections, no matter what a person's age. • Older individuals with memory loss should always be medically evaluated.
• Sleep patterns in older adults are characterized by less deep sleep and frequent arousals.	• Sleep medications should be avoided or used only when absolutely necessary. They are not well tolerated by older people. • Some suggestions to assist the person in getting a good night's sleep: (1) Eliminate caffeine drinks in the afternoon and evening. (2) Play soft music and have a warm beverage to help induce sleep. (3) Do not allow daytime napping to exceed 2 hours. (4) Exercise daily, but do so earlier in the day and not before bedtime. (5) Take a warm bath before bedtime. (6) A back rub or a foot massage before bedtime may promote sleep by helping the individual relax.

Adapted from Richman & Glantz, 1992a.

Table 11. Musculoskeletal changes and ways to help

Musculoskeletal changes	Ways to help
• Bone loss begins at 40 years of age and is greater in women. Muscle strength and function decrease with loss of muscle mass. Bones become more porous. There is an increased risk of fractures.	• Bone loss can be reduced with moderate exercise just three times a week. Weight and strength training can increase muscle mass in older individuals, even those past 80 years. Regular exercise can help maintain bone density. The best choice is weight-bearing exercise, such as walking or running.
• Trunk becomes shorter as a result of intervertebral space narrowing. Bone joints are less mobile. Posture becomes more stooped.	• Osteoporosis and osteoarthritis are two common skeletal and joint diseases seen in older people. Exercise helps joints to be more flexible and improves posture.

Adapted from Richman & Glantz, 1992a.

Module 2

Communicating Effectively

Goal:

To improve learners' communication with supervisors and clients

Objectives:

1. To define the components of basic communication
2. To list factors that promote good communication between worker and supervisor
3. To learn and practice active listening skills

Key Terms

Active listening: Listening skills that allow the listener to better understand what is being said by the speaker and that show the speaker that the listener cares and is truly listening to what has been said.

Communication: The act of sending and receiving information, thoughts, and feelings.

Invalidate: To make a person feel unimportant.

Nonjudgmental: An uncritical and fair attitude.

Paraphrase: To rephrase something that has been said.

Passive listening: Listening without seeming interested in what a speaker has said and without checking to confirm the speaker's meaning.

Platitude: A positive phrase or expression that has been used so often that it has become dull or meaningless.

Restate: Repeating what was said or in another way.

The ability to communicate effectively may be the most important skill that a care provider can learn. Their work with older people consists primarily of performing tasks, but it also includes establishing positive relationships. The care provider often must communicate why a certain task needs to be done, or she may need to coax the older person to help with the task. The care provider may also communicate her concern—or frustration—in nonverbal ways. Communication with the client's family may involve the reasons that the care provider cannot do certain tasks the family wants, or the need to encourage the family to offer more assistance.

COMMUNICATION IN THE WORKPLACE

Good communication is essential in the worker–supervisor relationship. A worker who knows what, how, and to whom she should report is an effective team member. When she hears the respect of her supervisor, she will feel better about the work she is doing.

Communicating, something that we all do every day, sounds easy, but it is actually a complicated process. There are three aspects of communication that we will concentrate on: how messages are sent and received, nonverbal communication, and active listening.

SEND A CLEAR MESSAGE

Communication is the successful transmission of information from one person to another—in other words, communication is a two-way street. The sender must send a message and the receiver must receive it in order for communication to take place. However, the communication is not successful unless the meaning of the message sent and the one received are the same. This is not an easy accomplishment. There are many points where something could go wrong. (See Figure 3 for a graphic depiction of the communication process.)

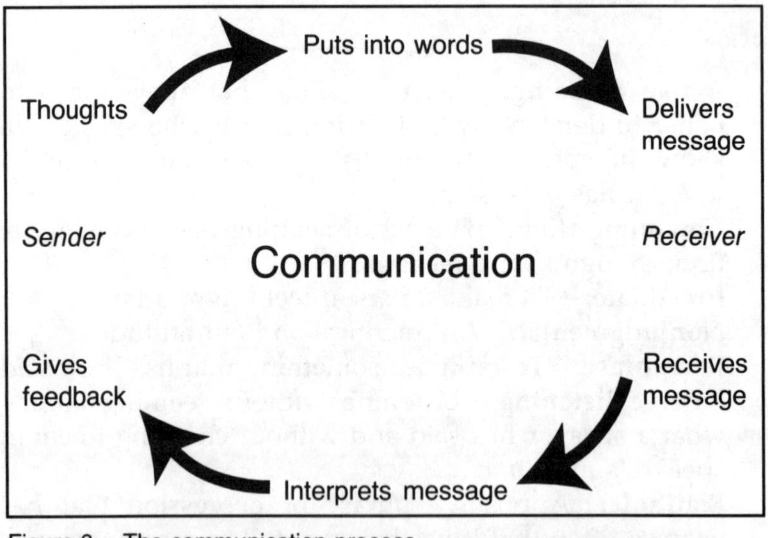

Figure 3. The communication process.

Problems in communication can begin before words are even spoken. We have all experienced times when our thoughts are unclear. Although we are not sure what we want to say, we say it anyway. The resulting confusion is no surprise.

DISCUSSION

Ask for examples of communication problems that learners have experienced with supervisors, with clients, and with clients' family members.

For example, a care provider may know that she is unhappy with her work, but she cannot explain why she is unhappy because she simply does not know. She could blame her supervisor. She could blame her clients. She could blame herself. In any case, she needs help sorting out her thoughts. We experience the same thing with our clients—they may not know where their anger is coming from. They just know that they are angry. They need help sorting things out.

We run into quite a few problems putting our thoughts into words. One major problem is that we often neglect to communicate at all. For many different reasons, we do not talk to each other, and the result is rarely good. When clear communication of expectations has not taken place, mistakes happen that could have been avoided. Care providers often have thoughts, feelings, and information that the supervisor should know about. When the care providers do not communicate with the supervisor, problems can occur. For example, a worker may feel angry because her supervisor has given her a very difficult client when she is feeling work-related stress or "burned out." The supervisor will not know how the worker is feeling unless she mentions it. Only then can she get the support she needs.

The care provider has unique insights into the needs of clients. Through her frequent interactions with the client she will see changes in behavior and the environment. For the team to be effective, the worker must make sure that she is providing as much detail as possible in her observations about the client to other members of the health care team. Observing and reporting are key aspects of the care provider's work. She is the eyes and ears of the family and of the employer.

TEST YOUR OBSERVATION AND REPORTING SKILLS

This activity demonstrates the importance of observing details about a client and reporting them clearly to a supervisor.

- Ask for a volunteer. You take the part of the worker, and the volunteer plays the supervisor. The "supervisor" asks for a status report on a client, Mrs. Rodriguez. The supervisor wants detailed information, but you answer questions in a vague manner: "She's fine, she ate well, but her sleep was restless."

- Ask participants what they thought about the report.
- Have another volunteer come to the front of the room and show how this type of reporting should be done.
- Ask for comments.

POSITIVE FEEDBACK

For some reason, many of us have a problem complimenting others and receiving compliments. We may be thinking a kind thought, but we do not put it into words. Unless the other person is a mind reader, it means nothing.

In *The One-Minute Manager*, Dr. Ken Blanchard suggests a new supervisory technique. He recommends that, rather than watching to see what people do wrong, supervisors should try to discover them doing something right and then pay them a compliment. This praise reinforces the correct behavior, shows that the supervisor is paying attention to the person, and enhances the worker's self-esteem (Blanchard & Johnson, 1983).

Blanchard's lesson is not just for supervisors. Workers need to learn it as well. Do you know how much a supervisor appreciates a compliment, and do you know how rarely she gets one?

✸ POSITIVE FEEDBACK

Have participants turn to the person who is sitting beside them and pay her a compliment about what she has said, what she is wearing, or her smile. Ask participants to think about how it feels to send and receive praise.

PUTTING THOUGHTS INTO WORDS

The message being sent often has more than one meaning, and the receiver must try to figure out what the sender *really* means. There are many common phrases and words that have a wide range of meanings. Ask the participants to put a numerical value on each of the following words and phrases: *often, occasionally, always, almost always, sometimes, seldom, never* (e.g., *often* = four times per week; *occasionally* = once per week). Misunderstanding simple words like these can cause problems. A client may want her bathroom cleaned "often." To her this means daily, but to the worker it means once per week. In this example, the client's anger and the worker's frustration may be avoided if the meaning of the word *often* is clarified.

✸ WORD MEANINGS

Ask how many times in a week participants go out to dinner if they go out *often*. How many times a week do they go out to eat if they go out *occasionally?* How many times a week do they go out to eat if they go out *seldom?* Ask participants to raise their hands if *often* means four or more times, three times, two, or one. Do the same for *occasionally* and *seldom*. You will see how people interpret these words differently.

There is not likely to be total agreement on many terms that we commonly use. We must be very careful that the understanding of the sender and the receiver are the same. Communication can be difficult when the message is not clear enough and when the person who receives the message does not ask for clarification.

TEARING A SHEET OF PAPER

- Ask for four volunteers. Tell them to come to the front of the room and face the group. Give each volunteer a piece of paper. Tell the volunteers that they must keep their eyes closed throughout the exercise and not ask questions.
- Tell volunteers to fold their paper in half and then tear off the bottom right-hand corner. Have them fold the paper again and tear off the upper right-hand corner. Finally, have them fold the paper in half again and tear off the top left-hand corner.
- Instruct the volunteers to unfold their papers, open their eyes, and show their papers to the audience. The papers will not all look the same.

Discussion Questions:

- What words in the directions could be interpreted in different ways?
- How could the directions have been better stated?
- What could the volunteers have done to clarify that they understood the message?

Adapted from Scannell, E., & Newstrom, J. (1983). *More games trainers play.* New York: McGraw-Hill. Reproduced with permission of McGraw-Hill.

MESSAGE DELIVERY

Any message can be delivered in a variety of ways. Comedians say that the success of a joke depends upon the delivery. Tone of voice, facial expressions, body language, and gestures all affect how a message is delivered. For example, tone of voice can make a profound difference in the way a message is sent. "Nonverbal communication" may also include eye contact, posture, and the distance between people.

WAYS OF COMMUNICATING

- Ask volunteers to repeat these phrases to the class, each using a different tone of voice. Discuss responses.

  - "That's OK; I'm not angry."
  - "I'm glad my mother-in-law is coming to dinner."
  - "No, I'm not busy."
  - "You were sick yesterday?"
  - "That is not my job."

- Ask for volunteers to act out a variety of messages without speaking.

a. Supervisor is sitting at desk while aide walks into the room.
   - Give the message that you are too busy to talk.
   - Give the message that you are bored by what is being said.
   - Give the message that you are very interested in what is being said.

b. A care provider is in a client's home when the supervisor comes for a home visit.
   - Worker shows anger and defensiveness toward supervisor.
   - Worker shows openness to supervisor's comments.

RECEIVING MESSAGES

Many factors can affect how a message is received. Hearing loss, medications, disabilities, and depression can have major effects on how a client receives a communication. Clients with hearing impairments need special attention. Figure 4 is a list of techniques to use to improve communication with these clients.

Stress and work load are factors that can affect how a worker—or a supervisor—hears messages from co-workers and clients. Also, a limited knowledge of English can be a substantial factor for both clients and care providers.

One reason that a message may not be received correctly is because of poor listening skills. It is interesting how little we are taught about how to listen. Yet listening is one of the most important factors in communication. There are some behaviors on the part of the receiver that make it hard to listen. When someone is listening to a message, he or she may be preparing responses instead of listening, thinking of other things, or feeling bored and uninterested in what is being said. Often, people will not completely attend to what is being said because they believe they already know the answer or their biases and stereotypes stand in the way of hearing new information. There are frequent distractions in the health care environment that make listening difficult, and concentration may be difficult due to fatigue or illness.

A poor listener shows inattention by various means. Some of the behaviors of a poor listener are not paying attention to the speaker, listening passively, preparing an answer to the speaker before she is through talking, rushing the speaker, interrupting the speaker or changing the subject, and becoming emotional. Another common mistake for a listener to make is to give

- Be sure you have the person's attention before beginning to speak.
- Face the person and stand reasonably close.
- Lower the pitch of your voice.
- Speak clearly and slowly.
- Use short sentences.
- Avoid background noise.
- Encourage the use of nonverbal communication, such as touch.
- Use written communication if you are unable to communicate verbally.
- Do not shout; shouting makes words less clear and may cause pain.
- Do not speak with something in your mouth or with your hands over your lips.
- Give clues about what is being discussed.
- State your name before making a statement or asking a question.
- Restate your sentence when you are not understood.
- Talk toward "better" ear, for many people hear better out of one ear.
- Recognize that illness or fatigue reduces the ability of a person with a hearing impairment.
- Do not exhaust the person with irrelevant noise or chatter.
- Visual cues may assist the client; use hand gestures when appropriate; provide the opportunity for lipreading.

Figure 4. Techniques to improve communication with clients who have hearing loss.

advice when it is not asked for. See Figure 5 for common barriers that poor listeners use to impede communication.

COMMUNICATION VIGNETTE

Read the following narrative to the group.

This is a story about a woman and her hard day. She got to work only to have her boss tell her that business has been so bad that he has to lay her off. She needs to clear out her desk and leave. He's sorry; after all, she's been with the company for eight years, but times are hard. All she'll get is 1 week's severance pay. When she gets home, she finds a number of unpaid bills. Some of them threaten to turn her over to a collection agency.

But that's not all! She goes into the kitchen and finds a note from her husband. He has decided to leave her and live with his 20-year-old secretary. His lawyer will be contacting her about the divorce. In tears and shock, she calls her best friend and tells her this story. Her friend says, "That job was awful anyway. And your husband, you're better off without the bum. But I know how you

CHANGING THE SUBJECT

It is often tempting to change a subject because the subject is uncomfortable. The client may be depressed and speaking about things that are discouraging to hear. Hang in there! He or she may need to talk about something that is deeply troubling. Changing the subject will not take the problem away, although listening may very well ease the load.

USING PLATITUDES

- "Oh, you'll get over it."
- "Just make the most of it."
- "Tomorrow's another day."
- "It's God's will."

We offer these words of encouragement from time to time, and, at some point in the conversation, these reassurances may be much appreciated. However, when a person comes to you with a problem, platitudes may completely invalidate his or her feelings. Platitudes may be useful at a later point in the conversation, after the individual has had the opportunity to air his or her feelings.

ASKING CLOSED-ENDED QUESTIONS (YES/NO)

Yes/no questions are useful when you want quick answers, not when you are actually interested in a conversation. Open-ended questions are far more likely to lead to interesting dialogue. For example:

Yes/No Questions	Open-Ended Questions
• "Do you need help?"	• "How may I help you today?"
• "Would you like to go outside?"	• "Where would you like to go?"

GIVING ADVICE

It is not our place to give advice or make recommendations. Just listening to our clients will usually help them to arrive at their own decisions.

TALKING ABOUT YOURSELF

Caregiver–client discussion is not restricted, but the caregiver's role is to listen to our clients, not to air our own problems.

SHOWING DISAPPROVAL AND PASSING JUDGMENT ON THE CLIENT

It is extremely important to remain nonjudgmental of clients. We have not walked in their shoes and cannot understand what their lives have been like.

ASKING "WHY" QUESTIONS

"Why" questions are a way of judging another person:

- "Why did you do that?"
- "Why are you thinking that?"

Figure 5. Barriers to effective communication.

feel. Let me tell you about *my* day." How do you think the woman felt toward her friend? What types of behaviors does the friend show? How could she have been a better listener?

EFFECTIVE LISTENING SKILLS

A person who is an effective listener shows positive behaviors. Paying attention to the speaker, adopting an accepting attitude, and allowing the speaker plenty of time are just a few ways to be an effective listener. Staying on the subject and being aware of your own emotional reactions to what is being said also help. Figure 6 summarizes the ways to listen effectively.

As you can see, the process of communication is very complicated. There are many points at which the message may be lost. The final factor in good communication is one that is often underestimated. That is when we "interpret the message" that has been sent. At this point, we develop our own understanding of what has been said. Active listening is a tool that will allow you to become very involved in the communication process. You can make sure that you understand not only what the speaker has said, but also how she feels. We do this by giving the speaker feedback about what we have heard. The speaker may then confirm or correct our understanding.

We often assume that we know what a person is saying without checking to make sure that we are correct. When we carefully listen, then check to see if we heard correctly, we are participating in active listening. Listening should not be a passive activity during which listeners simply sit and hope that they understand what is being said. There are too many points along the way during which the message may go wrong. Active listeners become very involved in the process, constantly checking to see if they are on target in what they understand. They practice active listening behaviors, as illustrated in Figure 7.

Paraphrasing what you heard means restating, in your own words, what the other person has said to check whether your understanding is correct. It also gives the speaker a chance to correct you if you have misunderstood. You might say such things as "Do you mean that . . . ?" or "I understand that you're saying . . . ."

- Pay attention to the speaker.
- Adopt an accepting attitude.
- Allow the speaker plenty of time.
- Stay on the subject.
- Be aware of your own emotional responses.
- Use active listening.

Figure 6. Effective listening skills. (From Steil, L. et al. (1983). *Effective listening: key to your success.* New York: McGraw-Hill; reprinted by permission.)

PARAPHRASE WHAT HAS BEEN SAID

Restating, in your own words, what the other person has said gives you a chance to check whether your understanding of what has been said is correct. It also gives the speaker a chance to correct you if you have misunderstood. You might say such things as "Do you mean that . . . ?" "I understand that you're saying . . ."

REFLECT THE SPEAKER'S FEELINGS

The feelings behind what is being said are often as important as the words, if not more so. Therefore, it is important to try to understand the underlying feelings, attitudes, beliefs, or values. You might make such statements as "That must have made you upset." "I imagine you were thrilled about that." "Does that worry you?"

ASK FOR MORE INFORMATION

We often need more information in order to understand what has been said. In most cases, we simply need to ask for clarification. Responses may include "I'm interested. Tell me more about that." "What happened after that?" "How did you feel when that happened?"

NONVERBAL COMMUNICATION

There are many ways through which the speaker can tell whether we are listening. Through our eyes, our posture, and our gestures, we communicate our interest in what is being said.

Figure 7. Active listening behaviors.

ACTIVE LISTENING

Choose three learners and give each one a slip of paper. Read each statement and read the possible responses. Ask which responses illustrate good or poor listening habits. Ask the group for other possible responses.

Statement: My daughter wants me to go in the nursing home.

A. Well, maybe you should consider it. Things are hard for you here.
B. How could she say that! After all you've done for her!
C. How do you feel about that?

Statement: I haven't been sleeping well lately.

A. Try some of these pills. They work great for me.
B. What's keeping you up?
C. Don't worry; you'll catch up on your sleep later.

Statement: I just can't handle this job anymore.

A. Is something at work bothering you today?

B. I know what you mean. I have this client who's driving me crazy!
C. The pay is terrible, and the hours are long; you should just quit.

Statement: My husband and I had a big fight last night.
A. Again? I don't know why you ever married him.
B. You're upset about the fight.
C. Every couple has fights. It's just part of marriage.

Statement: I've been a nervous wreck lately.
A. I'm not surprised. You're always trying to do too much.
B. Tell me about it! I've been feeling frazzled too.
C. What's going on that makes you feel that way?

Statement: Sometimes I feel like I'm of no use to anybody anymore.
A. Oh, no! You're a wonderful person!
B. It sounds as if you're feeling down today.
C. Well, it's not going to do you any good to feel sorry for yourself.

When an active listener reflects the speaker's feelings, she comments on the feelings behind what is being said, and these feelings can be as important as the words, if not more so. Understanding the underlying feelings, attitudes, beliefs, or values of a statement is useful for a care provider who is creating a successful relationship. Statements such as "That must have made you upset," "I imagine you were thrilled about that," or "Does that worry you?" tell the person you are talking with that you care and that you are paying attention.

We often need more information in order to understand what has been said. In most cases, we simply need to ask. Your question elicits more information from the speaker and gives him or her the opportunity to expand on the thought. In this way the listener can learn more about the problems, concerns, fear, or joys of the speaker.

Module 3

Understanding and Identifying Depression and Recognizing the Risk of Suicide

---

Goal:

To describe the signs of depression and ways the care provider can help the depressed older person

Objectives:

1. To understand the prevalence and severity of depression in older people
2. To recognize the signs and symptoms of severe depression in older people
3. To identify the changes in the older person's behavior that are the warning signs of depression
4. To recognize the potential for successful treatment of an older person's depression
5. To learn to cope with the stress involved in working with a depressed client

Key Terms

Empathy: Understanding and sensitivity toward the feelings of others.
Depression: A medical problem often caused by illness, medication, or chemical changes in the body.
Stress: A physical, chemical, or emotional factor that causes bodily or mental tension.
Suicidal: Having the impulse to kill oneself.

People mean many different things when they use the word *depression*. Depression is used to describe a range of conditions from the low feelings experienced at times by everyone to severe clinical depression. The different types of depression are distinguished by their severity.

THE DIFFERENT TYPES OF DEPRESSION

The mildest form of depression refers to the kind of "up-and-down" feelings that everyone experiences. These are the kind of low feelings that can be caused by a reprimand from a supervisor, an argument with a spouse, or a hard day at work. "Up-and-down" describes a mood that is a temporary reaction to stress, tension, or disappointment. When people are feeling this type of depression, they usually say, "Oh, I've just got the blues," "I'm feeling kind of down today," or "I'm just down in the dumps." The "up-and-down" type of depression comes and goes by itself and is a normal part of living.

The word *depression* is also used to describe the kind of emotions people feel following a loss. This is the type of depression people experience when they are grieving, and it often takes quite a while before it goes away. Because of the many losses they experience, older people often have this kind of depression. It is a normal reaction to the loss of a job, the loss of a friend, or the death or illness of a loved one.

The third kind of depression, clinical depression, is very serious and does not represent a normal part of life or a normal part of aging. Clinical depression is a medical illness that makes people feel hopeless and burdened, as if they were carrying around a sack of bricks. No matter how much they try, they are unable to shake off the condition. Left untreated, this kind of depression can have very serious consequences, affecting the way a person feels, thinks, and behaves. It can even affect a person's physical health.

Depression, ranging from mild to severe, affects many older people. "Among persons in the community, between 1 and 2 percent suffer a major or clinical depression. Dysthymic disorder, a more chronic and milder form of depression, is found among an additional 2 percent" (Blazer, 1990). The incidence of depression is found more often in older people who are physically ill or in institutions. "Among the medically ill and persons in long-term care facilities, clinical depression is found in about 12 to 16 percent, with an additional 20 to 30 percent suffering appreciable depressive symptoms" (Blazer, ibid).

Depression can cause severe disability and even death. For older people, it is particularly worrisome, because it can cause them to stop eating and starve to death; to stop taking care of their health, causing serious physical problems; to stop taking medications, including lifesaving medications for such problems as heart disease and hypertension; or to commit suicide.

People with depression experience a narrow range of emotions. Their affect (facial expression, tone of voice, etc.) is flat. They rarely show any joy or take pleasure in anything taking place around them.

SIGNS AND SYMPTOMS OF DEPRESSION

People who are depressed show signs of feeling extremely sad, worthless, or hopeless. They may become forgetful or seem unfocused. They can become angry easily or are constantly irritable. Anxiety is another sign of depression. Also, depressed people often express feelings of guilt. Figure 8 is a comprehensive list of symptoms caused by depression.

People suffering from clinical depression are unable to enjoy any aspect of their lives and have great difficulty focusing or paying attention. Older people often do not complain about being depressed, but they do frequently complain about things that can add up to depression. Many older people have physical problems, but people who are preoccupied with their physical illnesses may be depressed. They may say things like "I don't know what's the matter with me. I just don't feel right." These complaints may be covering up their depression.

Depression can also affect the way a person thinks. Depressed people can have false beliefs about themselves. They often believe they are worthless and that nothing they do is right. Depressed people can be irritable, disagreeable, and at odds with everything.

People with depression think nothing will ever get better, and they are overwhelmed by guilt. They put themselves down and cannot see anything good about themselves. A depressed older person may have difficulty paying attention and also may be forgetful.

FEELINGS CAUSED BY DEPRESSION

- Extreme sadness
- Hopelessness
- Worthlessness
- Inability to enjoy life

NEGATIVE THOUGHTS CAUSED BY DEPRESSION

- Fear nothing will ever get better
- Overwhelming guilt
- Low self-esteem
- Difficulty in paying attention
- Forgetfulness

BEHAVIORAL CHANGES CAUSED BY DEPRESSION

- Excessive crying
- Slowness in walking, talking, and moving
- Low energy
- Poor personal appearance
- Jittery, unsettled manner
- Anxiety
- Excessive anger
- Sleep disorders

PHYSICAL CHANGES CAUSED BY DEPRESSION

- Too much or too little appetite
- Weight loss
- Headaches, shortness of breath, stomachaches

SUICIDAL TENDENCIES CAUSED BY DEPRESSION

- Thoughts about wanting to kill oneself
- Suicide
- Suicide attempts

Figure 8. Signs of depression checklist.

DEPRESSION IS DIFFERENT FROM DEMENTIA

Sometimes an older person's forgetfulness and difficulty in concentrating are mistakenly assumed to be Alzheimer's disease or some other type of dementia. However, an older person who begins to forget and experiences other symptoms of dementia may be depressed. Unfortunately, it can be very difficult even for an experienced clinician to tell the difference between depression and dementia. This is particularly true because the awareness of early dementia may cause a person to become depressed.

Both depression and dementia have the following similarities:

- Changes in sleep patterns
- Appetite changes
- Fatigue
- Behavioral slowing or agitation
- Complaints of diminished ability to think or concentrate

In addition, people suffering from either depression or dementia may become careless in their grooming. The decreased variation in facial expression in dementia may be interpreted as the loss of interest or pleasure seen in depression. However, several clues may help the worker distinguish between the two conditions. Depressed older adults tend to complain about memory difficulties, even though they do not show any significant memory loss. Conversely, people with mild dementia show clear signs of memory loss but usually overestimate their own memory ability. Depressed older people may have a difficult time remembering neutral or positive experiences when they can easily remember negative events (Birren & Schaie, 1990). A person suffering from depression related to dementia can and should be treated for depression. If the care provider suspects either dementia or depression, a medical diagnosis and treatment should be sought.

Because older people often do not complain about feeling depressed, the care provider needs to be aware of *behavioral changes* that may suggest a depressed client. People who are depressed often cry a lot; may neglect their appearance; and may walk, talk, and move slowly.

Depression may also cause physical changes. A depressed person can have sleep disorders; eat too little or too much; lose or gain weight inexplicably; and experience headaches, shortness of breath, stomachaches, and other physical ailments.

Depression is a serious illness, and care providers working with older clients must be able to recognize its symptoms. A useful checklist of symptoms from the Public Health Service may help in determining whether a client is depressed (National Institutes of Health, 1994). Symptoms can include the following:

- Persistent sad or "empty" mood
- Loss of interest or pleasure in ordinary activities, including sex
- Decreased energy, fatigue, being "slowed down"
- Sleep disturbances, insomnia, early-morning waking or oversleeping
- Eating disturbances (loss of appetite and weight, or weight gain)

- Difficulty concentrating, remembering, making decisions
- Feelings of guilt, worthlessness, helplessness
- Thoughts of death or suicide, or suicide attempts
- Irritability
- Excessive crying
- Chronic aches and pains that do not respond to treatment

Not every depressed person will exhibit all of these symptoms. However, the more of these symptoms the person shows, the greater the chance that he or she is depressed. Perhaps the most important of these symptoms are crying easily or spontaneously, and waking up early in the morning.

Care providers should be aware if a client experiences either of these symptoms. If depression is suspected, the care provider should notify a supervisor so that family members can be notified and arrangements for medical diagnosis and medical help can be made.

Physical and Visual Clues

Depression interferes with an older person's daily functioning and activities. Often a depressed person is not concerned about personal appearance and neglects hair, teeth, and skin care. A depressed person may look sad without complaining about being sad. Depression may also cause a person to want to stay in bed more than is normal (see Figure 9).

Caregivers are often the only people who see these older persons regularly. They have the opportunity to observe clients closely over time. This activity is an important part of their job. Being able to identify signs of depression and knowing when to report changes in behavior to a supervisor are cru-

- Depressed people may not take care of their hair, teeth, and skin. When questioned, they will not seem to care how they look or will say, "Oh, I just don't have the energy to do it."
- Depressed people may look sad even though they do not complain about being sad. They may cry a lot for no reason or because of sad things that happened many years ago.
- Depressed people may suddenly look old. When you try to remember what the person was like 6 months or 1 year ago, you are amazed when you realize how much he or she has aged in a short time. This is an important sign because people do not really age that much in 6 months or even 1 year unless they have had physical problems.
- Depressed people may want to stay in bed all the time.
- Depressed people may withdraw from activities or seem to be just going through the motions. The person does not seem to enjoy anything anymore.
- Depressed people may talk about wanting to commit suicide or say, "It would be just as well if I were hit by a car."

Figure 9. Observations of a depressed person.

cial skills. Many symptoms of depression are the same as symptoms of other serious problems: dementia, malnourishment, medication misuse, or alcoholism. A trained, skilled caregiver will know what is normal for the older person and can identify changes. Use Figure 9 as a guide when discussing case examples or vignettes with the group.

CASE STUDY

Read the following case study aloud to group participants and then discuss it.

Mrs. Stone has stopped taking care of her hair and skin, and no longer puts in her dentures each morning. When questioned about her personal hygiene, she responds, "I don't have the energy to make myself up!" She rejects the care provider's offers to go for a walk, claiming that she is too exhausted to get out of bed. The care provider notices that Mrs. Stone looks much older than she did 6 months earlier and that she spends a lot of her time crying for no apparent reason.

- How should the care provider interpret Mrs. Stone's behavior?
- What should she do?
- Ask participants for other case examples.

CAUSES OF DEPRESSION

Depression in older people can be caused by a variety of factors. Sometimes, people have a lifelong tendency toward depression. It becomes obvious only later in life when triggered by difficult circumstances, such as a chronic illness or the death of a spouse.

Sometimes a physical illness can cause depression by altering chemicals in the brain. Diabetes, hypothyroidism, kidney and liver dysfunction, stroke, heart disease, and infections can all cause depression. High blood pressure and Parkinson's disease medication, as well as some tranquilizers, sedatives and anti-inflammatory medication, can have depression as a side effect. The symptoms may show up immediately or not until after several months of taking the medication.

TREATMENT FOR DEPRESSION

Fortunately, in most cases depression can be treated. In fact, depression is one of the most treatable illnesses of older adults. Depression can be treated in three different ways: with medication; with "talk therapies," such as psychotherapy; and with electroconvulsive (shock) therapy.

Antidepressant medication can be extremely effective in treating the symptoms of severe depression, such as loss of energy, inability to enjoy things, and sleep and appetite problems. These medications work by bringing the relevant chemicals in the brain back into balance. People suffering from frequent depression may require ongoing medication to alleviate their depression. Others respond to antidepressant medication within 2–6 weeks.

Counseling or psychotherapy is generally used with moderate depression. When used with antidepressants, counseling can help the older person with problems of low self-esteem to develop better coping skills.

Electroconvulsive therapy (sometimes called "shock treatment") can be a safe and effective way to treat the severely depressed person who has not responded to other forms of treatment. It is used primarily in life-threatening situations in which the older person could starve to death or commit suicide. A pulse of electricity passes through electrodes on a person's scalp, producing changes in the brain. Although this therapy can help a severely depressed person feel better quicker than other treatments, it is generally not tried until other treatments have failed.

UNTREATED DEPRESSION IN OLDER PEOPLE

Although depression in older people responds well to treatment, it often goes untreated. Depression goes undiagnosed in older people for a variety of reasons. Some people, including older people themselves, believe that sadness and depression are a natural part of aging. Care providers should know that sadness and depression are not natural parts of aging. Clinical depression is not the result of growing old. It does not happen to all older people. Even people with chronic illness, financial problems, or other difficulties should not suffer from depression.

Another reason that depression is often misdiagnosed is that many people, including older people themselves, are not able to recognize the signs and symptoms of the disease. Physical illness can mask depression, and depression, in turn, can look like a physical illness.

Older people may also deny being depressed, because they feel that admitting to the feelings of depression is a sign of weakness. They may fear being labeled as weak or even crazy. Many older people were raised during a time in which it was not socially acceptable to be depressed. Old attitudes hang on and can prevent many older people from coming to terms with the fact that they have a debilitating and even life-threatening illness.

Some clients find it normal to talk about physical illness and express physical pain, but not to express emotional pain. They may somaticize, or give physical characteristics, to their depression. Headaches and stomachaches will be treated instead of the depression that brings these symptoms on.

Depressed people often drink heavily in an attempt to relieve depression, but heavy drinking can make depression worse. The use of drugs can also cause depression. Often, people abuse drugs to try to relieve their symptoms.

DEPRESSION AS A CAUSE OF DIFFICULT BEHAVIOR

It can be hard for a care provider to decide whether a client is just being difficult or is suffering from depression. These three questions may help identify the problem:

1. Has the person changed dramatically?
2. Has the change been constant for 2 weeks or longer?
3. Is the change interfering with the person's day-to-day functioning?

If the answer to all three questions is "yes," then the person may be depressed (Schmall & Stiehl, 1990).

If depression is suspected, the care provider should tell a supervisor. Friends and family members of the client should be asked if they have noticed changes in the client's mood. The three questions listed above are useful in this context also.

When working with the client, do not tell the client to "shape up" or to "snap out of it," or ask "what's wrong with you?" Do not be critical of the client's new behavior, difficult as it may be to deal with. Instead, suggest that the client consider seeing a doctor for a medical evaluation. It is important to rule out a physical illness or the side effects of medication.

Most depressed people will resist the suggestion that they are depressed. How does the care provider deal with a depressed client who resists help? It is important for care providers to talk with the client about specific physical changes, specific problems, false beliefs the client may have about depression and treatment, and the person's fears. Figure 10 is a list of issues that can be addressed.

The depressed person should be told about the care provider's concerns, but not in such a way that would make the person feel worse. Depressed clients should not be made to feel that they are being blamed. Talk to the client about recent changes, such as weight loss or gain, loss of energy, sleep disruption, or excessive crying. Other changes that should be discussed are not paying bills, not going to church, not wanting family and

- Specific physical changes you noticed
- Weight loss or gain
- Loss of energy
- Sleeping too much or not enough
- Crying a lot
- Not paying bills
- Not going to church (if client is a churchgoer)
- Not wanting family and friends to visit
- Not wanting to talk on the phone
- Not going out for walks
- Fears and false beliefs
- Fear people will think they are crazy
- Fear they will be locked up
- Old versus modern ideas about depression

Figure 10. Subjects to talk about with a depressed person.

friends to visit, not wanting to talk on the phone, and not wanting to leave the house.

A trained worker can explain to the client that depression is a medical problem often caused by illness, medications, or chemical changes in the body. She can reinforce that depression does not imply weakness or insanity. It is an illness that needs treatment, and it may not simply go away by itself.

A care provider should not promise clients that they will not be hospitalized, but should let them know that most depressed people are treated on an outpatient basis. Never threaten clients with institutionalization. This will not cause them to "snap out of it" and may cut off an important line of communication.

It is important for the care provider to avoid blaming the client. Recognize that depressed people are often unable to control the way they feel or behave. This may be difficult for the worker who believes that if the older person just tried harder, he or she would be fine! A care provider's attitude toward depression will affect the way she talks with the older person. A solid understanding of the relationship with the client will also influence her work. The care provider may not respond to a client's worries in an empathic way if she believes her job is to try to cheer the person up.

FOCUSING ON THE CLIENT

Read the following scenario to the group.

Mrs. Barnes has not been sleeping well. In the morning, her care provider, Carolyn Turner, tells her, "Mrs. Barnes, you know you shouldn't stay up all night. No wonder you feel so bad all day. You're not getting enough sleep! I can't believe you haven't seen a doctor yet. What's the matter with you?"

Has Carolyn Turner dealt with her client appropriately? How might she have approached the client differently? Ask for suggestions. Try to get learners to see that by using "I" statements rather than "you" statements, Ms. Turner could have shown her client that she is concerned about her. "I" statements tell the person that you care by sharing your feelings and the specific changes you observed without telling the person that she has done something wrong.

- Which is the better way to tell the person that you are concerned?
  - A. You mean you haven't seen your doctor yet?
  - B. I am concerned about you. May I help you call your doctor to make an appointment?
- Which is the better way to tell the older person that you care?
  - A. I've noticed lately that you are not sleeping well.
  - B. You haven't been sleeping lately!
- Discuss responses with the group.

The activity on client-focused communication shows that even the most well-meaning people may make comments or ask questions that do not enhance communication. Professional care providers are likely to talk with a depressed person regularly, and this is not an easy thing to do. The care provider should be alert for ways to open up communication with a depressed person.

The care provider should listen with empathy to a depressed client. Depressed people need someone to talk to who will listen and understand. Empathy involves being able to look at the world through the other person's eyes. Care providers need to communicate in a way that shows they have understood how the depressed person feels and the experiences behind these feelings.

Getting the person to talk and listening carefully to what the person says can offer the client hope. Reassure depressed clients over and over that the reason they feel so bad could be depression. Although depressed clients will say that they do not believe things will get better, they still need to hear that there is hope. Figure 11 offers guidelines for helping alleviate clients' fears.

A care provider's job is to help the person do things that she may no longer be able to do for herself. However, this increased dependency may be a factor behind the depression! A worker should encourage an older person to use her remaining capabilities. A client can be involved in tasks if activities are structured in small, simple steps so that the client does not feel overwhelmed. Emphasize doing things *with* clients rather than doing things *for* them. Doing everything for someone who is depressed can increase the person's feelings of helplessness and inadequacy.

A client who feels out of control can be rigid and uncooperative. There are often ways to regain control. The care provider can allow the client to make some decisions about what to eat, when to bathe, and what activities to do. However, avoid giving depressed people too many choices. They may feel overwhelmed and unable to choose. A choice between two simple items is best. Instead of "What would you like for lunch?" ask "Would you like tomato soup or a tuna sandwich for lunch?" When looking in the closet, ask "Would you like to wear the blue dress or the red one?"

The older person has the right to privacy and autonomy, including the right to make a bad decision. A worker may have a hard time watching a client do something that seems clearly incorrect. However, the best way to intervene is to share one's observations and concerns. The decision rests with the client.

Most importantly, a worker must be watchful for signs of suicide. The care provider is in a unique position. She can be the eyes and ears of the family and the employer. It is imperative that she be able to recognize changes in the older person and know when to report them.

DEPRESSION AS A PRELUDE TO SUICIDE

No one has to remain depressed. An older person does not have to be sad. It is important for the care provider to be aware of the signs and symptoms of clinical depression. Without treatment, clinical depression can kill.

Clinical depression makes everything seem depressing. People who are depressed lose their ability to imagine a time when things were good, and they

- Listen with empathy.
- Offer hope. Get the person to talk, and listen carefully to what the person says. Reassure the person over and over again that the reason he or she feels so bad is due to a medical depression that will end. Even though the depressed person will tell you that he or she does not believe things can get better, the need for hope is extremely important.
- Encourage physical activity, but do not push! For example, if a female client used to enjoy taking walks, do not expect her to initiate a walk. You will need to go and get her coat, hold it up as though you were helping her to put her coat on, and tell her, "Let's go outside for a walk." If she resists and says she cannot, you might suggest she try a short walk. Tell her that if she cannot tolerate the walk, you will be there to bring her back.
- Structure activities. Make things the person used to enjoy simpler to do. Encourage the person to do what he or she feels able to do. Be careful: Do not overwhelm the person by demanding more than he or she is able to do.
- Lighten the guilt. Recognize that depression is not something the person can change simply by being told to "shape up." Point out the person's strengths and the positive things she has done in her life before becoming depressed. When possible, identify specific positive things happening in the client's life in spite of the depression—for example, taking care of children, going to the doctor for help, making phone calls when upset, getting dressed, putting on makeup, asking for help with things difficult to do because of the depression.
- Emphasize doing with, rather than doing for. Doing everything for someone who is depressed can increase the person's feelings of helplessness and inadequacy.
- Restore areas of control. In many ways, rigidity and noncooperation are often an expression of the ways the depressed person is attempting to regain control over her life.
- Set limits. This is an act of caring that protects both you and the other person.
- Reminisce about positive past experiences. Ask direct questions about the past. Use old photos, scrapbooks, and other things from the past to help the person remember. Reminiscing may help the person to recall the past more positively and feel less worthless. Caution: When seriously depressed, some people cannot use reminiscing to feel better. If your client recalls only the pain, do not pursue this option.
- Respect the person's rights to privacy and autonomy. This includes the right to make the wrong decision.
- Be watchful for signs of suicide.

Figure 11. Ways to help a depressed person.

cannot imagine that things will ever get better. This is what is meant by the sense of hopelessness that they feel. These feelings are always present and may last for 2 weeks or longer. During this time, depressed people feel that nothing can help pull them out of their situation. Older people often talk about dying, but people who talk about wanting to die as a solution to their problems may be suicidal.

SUICIDE AND OLDER PEOPLE

Suicide is often associated with teenagers, or younger people in general. In fact, suicide is more common in older white men than in any other age group. Suicide is one of the leading causes of death among older adults, yet it is the leading cause of preventable death in this population.

When depression becomes severe, older people sometimes think about killing themselves, threaten to kill themselves, or actually kill themselves. People who are depressed may feel so bad that they believe their pain can only be relieved by death. Of those who try to kill themselves, more older people will be successful in their attempt than any other age group; in fact, they account for more than 25% of the suicides committed (Billig & Nathan, 1987). The threat of suicide in a depressed older person should always be taken seriously.

Suicide Warning Signs

There are usually warning signs when a depressed person is considering suicide. Some people talk about their plan. Others behave in certain ways. (See Figure 12 for a detailed list of key behaviors.)

An older person who is depressed and feels the situation is hopeless is at risk for suicide. He or she may talk about wanting to commit suicide to "relieve the pain" or to "solve my problems." This kind of statement should never be taken lightly or brushed off. Responding to such a statement in a way that opens communication is helpful to the client. Another sign of suicidal ideas is unusual behavior on the part of the depressed person—a sudden or dramatic

- The older person is depressed and feels his or her situation is hopeless.
- The older person talks about wanting to end his or her life to "relieve the pain" or "solve my problems."
- The older person describes the method of suicide.
- Unusual behavior appears that is a sudden or dramatic change.
- The older person has a specific plan for suicide—the more specific the plan, the higher the risk.
- The odds are high that the suicide method the older person uses will result in his or her death.
- It is easy for the older person to obtain the means for suicide—gun, pills, car—the easier this is, the higher the risk.
- The older person becomes isolated—when a depressed, suicidal person avoids others, the risk is greater.

Figure 12. The warning signs of suicide.

change, when the client does not act normally. Sudden happiness after a serious depression is also a clue that a person may be suicidal.

Depressed people who are suicidal are at particular risk when they have a specific plan: the more specific the plan, the higher the risk. With an older person, the odds are high that the person will be successful. Suicide attempts are not attention-getting devices. They are serious. A factor to consider when assessing risk is the access to the means (gun, pills, car) to carry out the suicide plan. Does the client have medication stored up? Is there a gun in the house? If a suicidal person is isolated or deliberately becomes isolated, he or she is at increased risk.

While some older adults attempt to commit suicide on the spur of the moment, they are more likely to be motivated to do so after the death of a spouse or when abusing alcohol and other drugs. The depressed person who experiences an upswing in mood may have come to a sense of peace regarding his or her death. This person may also be making plans for giving away possessions or cleaning up personal affairs to avoid leaving a mess for the family. When the depressed person is coming out of a depression, observers may think the worst has passed. This is a time for increased watchfulness. Holidays and anniversaries are especially hard times for depressed, suicidal older people. Even the depressed person who has dementia (severe memory loss) should be considered at risk.

A provider should always take suicide threats seriously. This is a time to let a client know that confidentiality may have to be broken. The care provider must follow the employer's suicide crisis plan, beginning with reporting the threats to a supervisor. Avoid judging, and never threaten institutionalization. The care provider is in the unique position of being able to show concern and empathy by listening to the depressed client. See Figure 13 for a model suicide-prevention policy.

- Always take a suicide threat seriously.
- When reporting, be sure to state the frequency of the threats, any recent changes in the client's behavior, whether the person has a plan, and whether the person has the means to fulfill the plan.
- Steps to take when reporting:
  √ Call supervisor.
  √ If the supervisor is not available, ask for the case manager.
  √ Report the threat to a family member.
- Call 911 if the client has attempted suicide or if such an attempt seems imminent.

Figure 13. Model suicide-prevention policy.

HELP OTHERS BY TAKING CARE OF YOURSELF

Working with depressed clients is very demanding. Because this work is so demanding and draining, it is important that care providers know how to take care of themselves. They need to avoid suffering from the same symptoms as their clients!

STRESS MONITORING

- Distribute handout "Are You Under Stress?"
- Allow 20–30 minutes for learners to complete the questionnaire.
- Discuss responses.
- Distribute handout "No One Is an Is-Land."
- Discuss the need for supports.

Because people are often unaware of their stress symptoms, it is a good idea for care providers to check their own stress levels periodically. Workers who experience any of the symptoms identified in the handout may be under stress and should consider methods of stress reduction.

Working with depressed clients who appear not to appreciate the care provider's help can be draining. One way workers can avoid becoming depressed is by understanding that their clients are not responsible for their behavior. Caregivers need to allow for this and be aware of their own feelings. They should set realistic expectations for themselves and appreciate the meaningful ways in which they are helping their clients. Recognizing their contribution can give them a better sense of self-esteem and pride.

"I KNOW"

The discussion of depression draws upon the care provider's personal experiences in coping with depression and in caring for depressed or suicidal patients. Because these problems can be depressing to talk about, a game (similar to the television show *Jeopardy*) can be played to review the material presented. The learner who wants to try to win a prize will need to listen carefully.

Materials needed:

- Watch with second hand
- Tally pad and pen
- Prizes

The game is played with three or more contestants. A Game Host should also be selected. The board is laid out with various categories relating to depression and suicide. Each category includes four questions that are worth from $100 to $400. Give a copy of the "Questions and Answers" handout to the Game Host. Contestants draw numbers to decide who starts. The first contestant chooses a category and a dollar amount. The Host reads a question, and if the contestant knows the answer she should hold up her hand. She will be given 5 seconds to answer the question. All answers must be phrased with "I know. . . ." If the contestant answers the question correctly, the dollar value will be credited to her account. If the answer is incorrect, the contestant "loses" that amount of money along with the turn. The contestant with the most money wins.

Table 12 contains all the questions and answers to the "I Know" game.

Table 12. "I know" questions and answers

Category: Kinds

$100 Q. Is the normal depression that is part of living best described as "ups and downs," "grief," or "depression the medical illness"?
A. Ups/downs

$200 Q. Can abusing alcohol cause depression?
A. Yes.

$300 Q. Can physical illnesses cause depression?
A. Yes.

$400 Q. Name the two symptoms that are the warning signs of depression as a medical illness.
A. Crying easily and early-morning waking.

Category: Symptoms

$100 Q. Name a feeling that is a symptom of depression.
A. Sad, hopeless, worthless, guilty, irritable, etc.

$200 Q. Name a physical complaint that is a symptom of depression.
A. Eat more/less, weight loss/gain, sleep more/less, etc.

$300 Q. Name a way a person behaves when depressed.
A. Cries a lot, does not take care of self, not much energy, etc.

$400 Q. Describe a way depression affects a person's thinking.
A. Forgetful, difficulty paying attention, thinks nothing will ever be better, puts self down, etc.

Category: Treatment

$100 Q. Describe a reason why an older person may not be treated for depression.
A. Attitudes—old people are sad, or are entitled to be depressed. No one recognizes symptoms, and it is hard to tell whether they are physical problems or depression.

$200 Q. Why may an older person be depressed?
A. Biological changes, any loss of something or someone important, reduced support system, physical illness, drugs, heredity, stress, personality.

$300 Q. Will depression as a medical illness go away with time?
A. No.

$400 Q. Can shock treatment help a depressed person feel better?
A. Yes.

Category: Risk Factors

$100 Q. Can a person die from an untreated depression?
A. Yes.

continued

Table 12. *continued*

$200 Q. Is a widow suicidal who says, "I can't wait to die so I can be with my husband!"
A. No.

$300 Q. Is an older woman suicidal when she says, "I'm tired of this pain. I'd rather be dead, and I'm going to walk in front a car some day."
A. Yes.

$400 Q. Can a depressed person who had memory loss be suicidal?
A. Yes.

Category: Ways To Help

$100 Q. What best conveys your concern when your client resists going to the doctor because of serious depression?
1. I am worried that you are not sleeping well. I think you need to see your doctor.
2. You shouldn't stay up all night. No wonder you feel bad; you're not getting enough sleep.

A. Statement 1.

$200 Q. Which statement is the best way to encourage your client to see her doctor?
1. You mean you haven't see your doctor yet?
2. I am concerned about you. I'll help you call your doctor.

A. Statement 2.

$300 Q. Which statement best tells the person that you understand?
1. You shouldn't feel that way. It's nothing to worry about. Lots of old people have a hard time. Stop feeling sorry for yourself.
2. You sound as if you're having a difficult time. You feel very afraid and ashamed.

A. Statement 2.

$400 Q. Which statement is the best way to encourage a depressed person to be physically active?
1. Get out of that chair; you need to go for a walk.
2. We are going for a walk; here is your coat.

A. Statement 2.

Module 4

Understanding Alzheimer's Disease and Other Dementias

Goal:

To increase learners' understanding of symptoms and behaviors of dementia

Objectives:

1. To describe Alzheimer's disease and other dementias
2. To learn symptoms and how to recognize them
3. To understand how the brain and nerve cells work
4. To describe how dementias are diagnosed

Key Terms

Dementia: A disease that causes a progressive deterioration in cognitive abilities and judgment.
Multi-infarct dementia (MID): Dementia due to repeated small strokes.
Senile: Exhibiting the characteristics of old age, especially a loss of mental faculties. Today we recognize that the forgetfulness and confusion previously called senility is not a normal part of aging.

At some point in time, most care providers will work with a client suffering from Alzheimer's disease or another dementia. It is crucial that the care provider understand these disorders.

SYMPTOMS OF DEMENTIA

Memory loss is just one symptom of dementia. Others include poor recall, reduced concentration, poor calculation, "tip of the tongue" phenomenon, date confusion, forgetfulness, poor hygiene, trouble learning new information, and difficulty completing old skills (Figure 14).

Most of us can remember being warmly greeted by a person who looked familiar but whose name we could not immediately remember. This is an example of poor recall, and the person with dementia frequently has these kinds of experiences.

The average adult can count aloud backwards from 100 by 7s. The first few digits are usually easy; after that, it becomes more difficult. A person with dementia has trouble with even the first few numbers.

The "tip of the tongue" phenomenon occurs when a person can visualize an object but cannot remember its name. The person knows that he or she knows the word or name, but cannot come up with it.

If a person shows up somewhere on the wrong date or shows up on the right date but at the wrong location, we say that the person is "confused on dates." This is a common occurrence among people with dementia.

The experiences of poor recall and concentration, calculation problems, "tip of the tongue" phenomenon, difficulty with new learning, and confused dates are signs that early Alzheimer's disease or another type of dementia could be occurring.

Besides those symptoms mentioned above, the following may also be experienced:

- Difficulty completing simple tasks, such as cooking or dressing
- Frequent forgetfulness
- Trouble remembering where to put things—for example, where does the carton of milk go after a glass is poured?
- Misplacing things that are regularly used (e.g., comb, toothbrush, or soap)
- Less concern with hygiene and grooming

Everyone forgets things at times—some of us more than others. Isolated instances of forgetting or misplacing things may not be cause for alarm. When these experiences occur frequently and together, however, they may be signs of serious memory loss.

Is memory loss normal? Is it inevitable? What makes it serious? This section examines dementia and Alzheimer's disease and examines the diagnosis of each. It also looks at how the brain works, because dementia is a disease of the brain. It provides a better understanding of some of the behaviors and characteristics of the client who suffers from one of these disorders.

At one time, senility was considered a normal part of aging, an understandable loss of mental faculties. Not long ago, when people reached old age and acted strangely, they were labeled "senile." This definition is no longer

- Poor recall
- Reduced concentration
- Ability to calculate decreases
- "Tip of the tongue" phenomenon
- Difficulty learning new concepts
- Confusion about dates
- Loss of old skills
- Increased forgetfulness
- Poor hygiene

Figure 14. Memory loss symptoms.

valid. These days, the term *senility* has been replaced by *dementia,* which means, literally, "away from the mind." Dementia is not the name of a disease. It refers to all of the diseases that cause memory loss and changes in personality and behavior. There are nearly 100 different diseases that cause dementia, and Alzheimer's disease is the most common.

The *DSM-IV* (American Psychiatric Association, 1994, p. 142) defines dementia as follows:

> A. The development of multiple cognitive deficits manifested by both
> (1) memory impairment (impaired ability to learn new information or to recall previously learned information)
> (2) one (or more) of the following cognitive disturbances:
> (a) aphasia (language disturbances)
> (b) apraxia (impaired ability to carry out motor activities despite intact motor function)
> (c) agnosia (failure to recognize or identify objects despite intact sensory function)
> (d) disturbance in executive functioning (e.g., planning, organizing, sequencing, abstracting)

THE VARIOUS TYPES OF DEMENTIA

There are two classifications of dementia: those that can be treated (reversible) and those that cannot be treated (irreversible). Some of the more common causes of reversible dementias are depression, infections, medication or drug-related problems, physical disease, stress, dehydration and nutritional deficits, and sensory problems (see Figure 15).

Depression is a treatable disease. Its early symptoms can look very much like those of Alzheimer's disease: poor concentration, forgetfulness, and poor hygiene. Thus, depression in older adults is often misdiagnosed as dementia. Moreover, many older people do not tend to seek treatment for depression; they view it as a weakness, not a disease.

Infections can also cause these symptoms. Fevers and urinary tract infections can influence the way older people behave.

DEPRESSION

- Early symptoms look very much like dementia: poor concentration, forgetfulness, poor hygiene.
- Often misdiagnosed as dementia.
- Often viewed as a weakness rather than a disease.
- Very treatable.

INFECTION

- Can cause symptoms similar to dementia.

MEDICATION OR DRUG-RELATED PROBLEMS

- Can cause symptoms similar to dementia.
- Older people metabolize medication differently than do younger people.
- Medication combinations can cause serious memory loss problems.

PHYSICAL DISEASE

- Insufficient blood supply to the brain, pain, and problems associated with illnesses can cause dementia-like symptoms.

STRESS AND GRIEF

- Stress or personal loss can affect the ability to function.

DEHYDRATION AND NUTRITIONAL DEFICITS

- Dehydration and nutritional deficits can cause dementia—for example, a reliance on coffee and canned soups and foods, both of which are diuretics, can cause the symptoms of dementia.

SENSORY PROBLEMS

- Sensory problems may mimic symptoms of dementia.
- Vision and hearing typically decline with age.

ALZHEIMER'S DISEASE

- Alzheimer's disease is the most common form of dementia.
- Alzheimer's disease causes brain damage and is terminal.
- Alzheimer's disease is not a form of mental retardation or mental illness.
- Alzheimer's disease affects personality, behavior, communication, and the ability to do things, as well as memory.

continued

Figure 15. Causes of dementia.

MULTI-INFARCT DEMENTIA (MID)

- The second most common form of dementia.
- Caused by multiple small strokes.
- Frequently occurs with Alzheimer's disease.

AIDS

- Dementia sometimes occurs in the late stages of AIDS.

CHRONIC ALCOHOL ABUSE

- Korsakoff's syndrome, caused by alcohol abuse, is a type of dementia.
- Symptoms may go away if the individual stops drinking, but there is a point at which chronic alcohol abuse causes permanent damage.

PARKINSON'S DISEASE

- Parkinson's disease may cause memory loss.

Figure 15. *continued*

Medication or drug-related problems that cause symptoms of dementia are common in older people. Many clients take several medications (both prescription and over-the-counter) simultaneously. Older people metabolize medication differently than do younger people. They frequently have more than one doctor—one for each problem—and do not tell one the medications that the others have prescribed. This situation can result in combinations of medications that cause serious memory problems.

Physical disease can cause mental change. An older person who has a heart attack (with no pain) may have symptoms of confusion because an insufficient amount of blood is reaching his or her brain.

Stress and grieving are often mislabeled as dementia or senility. Sickness, stress, feeling blue, fatigue, distraction, and/or suffering losses all affect one's ability to function.

Dehydration and nutritional deficits can cause dementia. For example, the older individual who drinks coffee and lives on canned soups and foods, all of which are diuretics, can become dehydrated and develop symptoms similar to dementia. The person who eats only prepared foods may suffer from vitamin deficiencies, which can also cause confusion.

Sensory problems may mimic symptoms of dementia. Vision and hearing typically decline with age. A woman who has substantial hearing loss or a recent widow living alone for the first time may misinterpret noises in the night as prowlers or burglars and may call the police frequently.

A second classification of dementias contains those that are irreversible and whose symptoms cannot be treated. These diseases usually get worse over time. Some common diseases of this type include Alzheimer's disease, Korsakoff's syndrome, Parkinson's disease, and acquired immunodeficiency syndrome (AIDS).

Alzheimer's disease is the most common form of dementia. Approximately 60% of all dementias are attributed to the disease. Although it is much more likely to strike older individuals, Alzheimer's disease can occur in middle age as well. Alzheimer's disease is a chronic, irreversible disease that causes damage to the nerve cells in the brain.

Alzheimer's disease is *not* a form of mental retardation or mental illness. Many people think of the disease as only a memory disorder, but it also affects personality, behavior, communication, and the ability to perform routine tasks.

Multi-infarct dementia (MID) and Binswanger's disease are also common causes of dementia. These diseases result from repeated transient ischemic attacks (TIAs), or small strokes. These strokes affect memory and communication, but rarely result in paralysis or muscle weakness, as most strokes do.

Chronic alcohol abuse (Korsakoff's syndrome) can cause dementia. If an individual stops drinking early enough, memory-loss symptoms may go away. However, there is a point at which chronic alcohol abuse causes permanent brain damage. At this point, even if the individual stops drinking, the disease will progress.

Parkinson's disease can sometimes result in symptoms of dementia. However, it is important not to confuse the Parkinson's patient's slowed reaction time and blank affect with dementia. Often, Parkinson's patients are alert and oriented, but appear demented because of these symptoms.

AIDS-related dementia may be caused by the human immunodeficiency virus (HIV) attacking the nervous system, with resulting damage to the brain and spinal cord. Signs of damage may include confusion, forgetfulness, indifference, and the inability to make decisions (Illinois Department of Public Health, 1983).

Alzheimer's Disease

Alzheimer's disease and other diseases that cause dementia are *not* normal parts of aging.

In the early stages of Alzheimer's disease, symptoms develop slowly and can go unnoticed by families and friends. The individual still has the ability to cover up mistakes. She may blame other people—"You were supposed to remind me of that appointment"—or make up excuses—"I no longer cook for myself; it's just too time consuming."

Occasional forgetfulness is not a symptom of Alzheimer's disease. Everyone forgets where glasses and keys are from time to time. Everyone sometimes does things that seem silly—like standing in the middle of a room trying to remember why one entered it in the first place. Alzheimer's disease has received so much attention that everyone over 65 who experiences forgetfulness thinks she or he has it. However, the disease is more complicated than that. Losing one's glasses all the time is not a cause for worry; forgetting that one wears glasses is sign of serious memory loss. Losing one's car keys is not a reason to worry; forgetting that keys are necessary to start the car is a sign of serious memory loss.

Alzheimer's disease progresses at a slow, steady rate. In the early stages of the disease the person may be able to function independently in most areas of life, requiring reminders and cues only. In the later stages of the disease the individual may require total assistance in all areas of care: feeding, dressing, grooming, and personal hygiene. However, not all people with Alzheimer's disease end their lives as bedridden, helpless people. If the individual is physically healthy, there is no reason why he or she should not remain ambulatory and at least marginally aware of his or her surroundings.

If an individual exhibits serious signs of memory loss, an evaluation and diagnostic workup are critical because some of the diseases that cause memory loss are treatable. Once the underlying disease is treated, memory improves.

The Diagnosis of Alzheimer's Disease There is currently no single test for Alzheimer's disease. The diagnosis is a process of elimination, as clinicians test for all possible illnesses and conditions that may cause dementia. If no other cause is found, then a "clinical diagnosis" of Alzheimer's disease is made. These tests have developed to such a sophisticated level that clinicians are correct in their diagnoses about 95% of the time. Brain biopsies are not done as part of the routine diagnosis because they are expensive, painful, and unreliable. At present, however, the only totally accurate way to determine whether an individual truly has Alzheimer's disease is through an autopsy.

The following are all part of the diagnostic evaluation process:

- **Physical exam/laboratory tests** (blood and urine) provide evidence of anemia or malnutrition.
- **Personal and family medical histories** can alert the doctor to exposure to chemicals, toxins, alcohol abuse, or relatives who may also have had dementia. Some researchers believe that Alzheimer's disease may have a genetic link.
- **Neurological exams** test for diseases of the nervous system, such as Parkinson's disease.
- **Psychological and psychiatric tests** check for personality disorders and psychiatric conditions.
- **Radiologic tests** (computerized axial tomography, CAT, and magnetic resonance imaging, MRI) rule out tumors, strokes, or disturbances in brain metabolism.

THE BRAIN

The brain is the body's control center. It controls thought, action, speech, and response. It controls behavior during anger, sadness, and apprehension. The brain also controls all of the 17 muscles necessary to swallow.

Different sections of the brain control different things. The **frontal lobe** (located in the front part of the brain; see Figure 16) is in charge of the ability to plan, behave, and respond emotionally. For example, in order to attend a funeral service, one plans how to get there, behaves respectfully, and responds emotionally to one's own pain and that of the family. Attention and concentration are also controlled by the frontal lobe.

The **temporal lobe** (located near the temple) controls communication. This includes the ability to talk, interpret what is being said and interpret nonlanguage sounds. The temporal lobe also controls the ability to use and understand words and pictures.

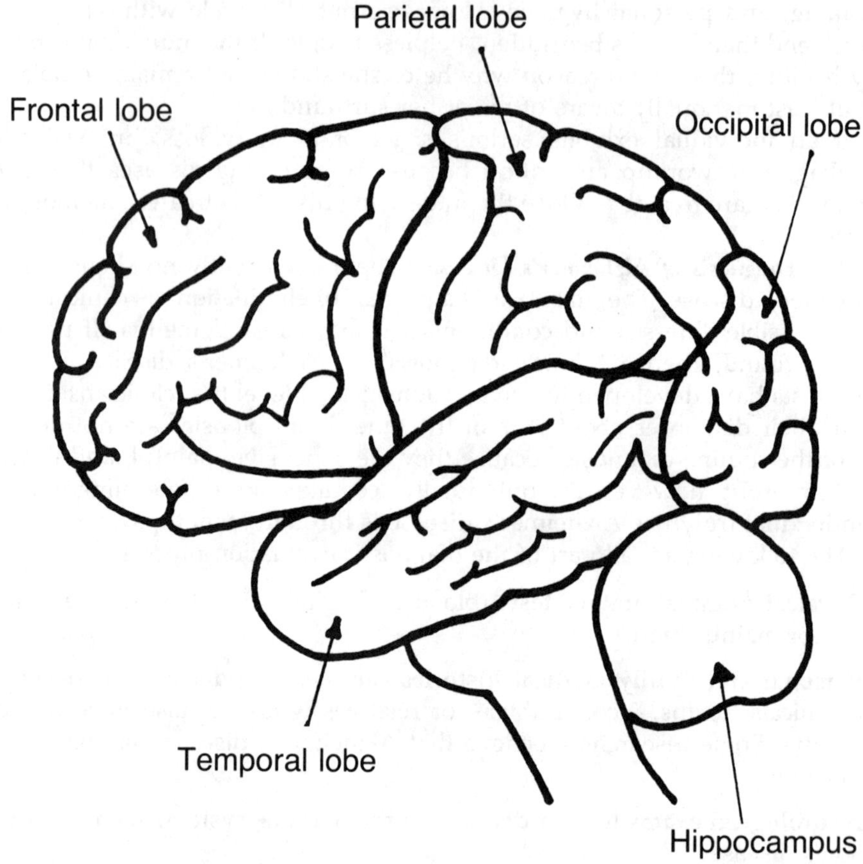

Figure 16. Segments of the brain.

The **parietal lobe** (located on the top of the brain) controls the body in space; for example, it directs how one sits on a chair. It helps one to see the world in three dimensions instead of two (flat) and gives information about the things in the environment.

The **occipital lobe** is located in the back of the brain. It is the vision-control center.

The **hippocampus** is underneath the brain and is where new information is stored and retrieved—in other words, "memory."

All of these areas of the brain are in constant communication with each other and the rest of the body. They do this through an intricate system of nerve cells. The brain has about 100 billion nerve cells, like the one seen in Figure 17. Nerve cells are continuously sending and receiving messages. This is a *very* simple explanation of what happens in your brain. At any given instant, there are many messages being sent simultaneously.

When an individual has Alzheimer's disease, there is damage to the brain. Little by little, the ends of the nerves die. Therefore, messages are not always sent. Some nerve cells can no longer "talk" to each other. The type of impairment is determined by which section of the brain is being affected by the disease process.

Nerve cells do not touch. They send messages to each other through chemicals. For example, one nerve cell uses a chemical messenger to tell another that the spherical, red object offered for dessert is an apple. In Alzheimer's disease there may not be enough of this chemical, or it may be missing. Therefore, some nerve cells do not get the message. When an individual with Alzheimer's disease sees an apple, messages may not be sent to all areas of the brain. The client may call it an apple, have memories of it, and realize it is near her, but she cannot plan how to use it. So she does nothing when she is told to "take a bite."

In addition to depleted or missing chemicals and dying nerve cells, the brain of the person with Alzheimer's disease can also develop plaques in the spaces between the nerve cells where the chemical should be. These plaques prevent messages from getting from one nerve cell to another.

The frontal lobe, which controls planning, is substantially impaired in someone with Alzheimer's disease. There are more dying nerve cells and plaques in this area. As a result, some people with Alzheimer's disease recognize their clothing but cannot put it on correctly. They may try to put their sweater on their legs or put their underwear over their pants.

Although the brain of a person with Alzheimer's disease is dying, individuals can still function with help. Sometimes all it takes is a reminder: "This is

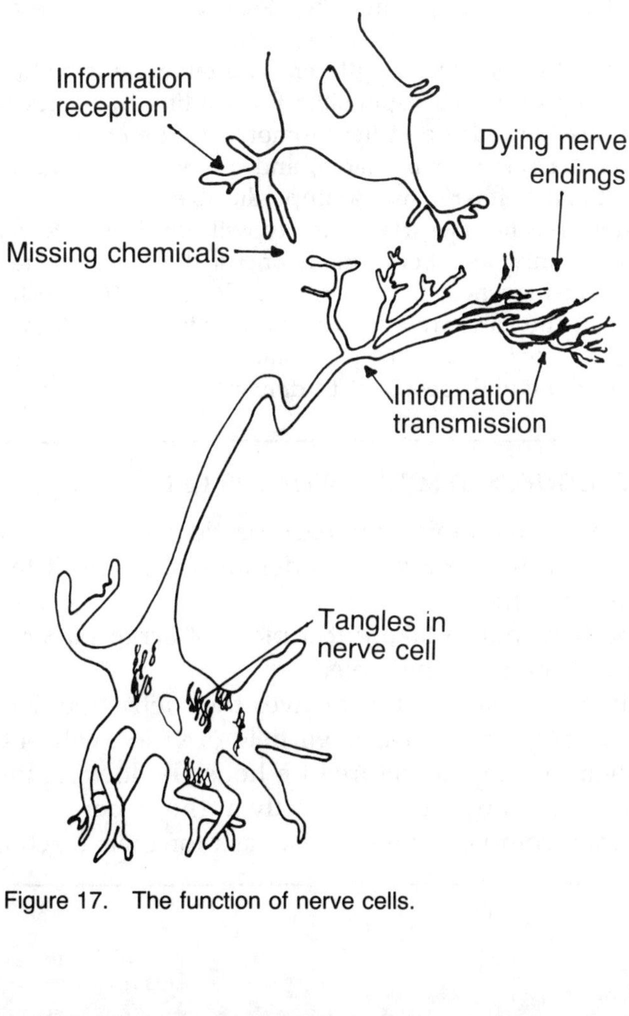

Figure 17. The function of nerve cells.

your sweater; let's put it on your arms." Or handing the client the apple and leading it to the mouth may remind the client to eat.

Individuals with this disease make many mistakes because of missing chemicals, plaques, and dying nerve cells. They may urinate in the wrong place, wear their clothing backwards, eat things that are inedible, or experience emotions that do not match the situation, all because of the destruction that Alzheimer's disease causes in the brain's nerve cells.

Imagine the frustration of seeing a comb and knowing it is something to use on your hair, but having no idea what to do with it. Imagine seeing a picture of a familiar and loved person, but having no idea what his or her name is. The impact of this disease upon an individual's emotional well-being is devastating.

There are a few things to remember that may help in working with a client who has Alzheimer's disease. Damage may occur in many different areas of the brain. If there are more patches of dying nerve cells in the temporal lobe, which is responsible for communication, the individual may have trouble talking and understanding spoken language. He or she may frequently experience "tip of the tongue" phenomenon, where a word is known but not easily recalled. If there are more patches of dying nerve cells in the parietal lobe, he or she may not be able to maneuver her body into a chair or out of the room. Changes in the floor or carpet may be perceived as holes because of perceptual problems.

Every individual is affected differently; interventions will differ according to the client. The chemical responsible for sending messages between nerve cells may be missing today and here tomorrow. Therefore, one day the client may recognize her caregiver by name, and the next she may not. This makes the person with Alzheimer's disease unpredictable. Avoid assuming that a person who cannot put her sweater on today will not be able to put it on tomorrow either. For family members, this is one of the most frustrating aspects of the disease. You may hear a spouse say, "You did this yesterday. What is wrong?" Part of the care provider's responsibility is to educate family members. The care provider can help families by demonstrating different approaches to working with people with dementia.

THE CONFUSED MIND—WHAT IS IT LIKE?

- Hand out a small mirror to each participant.
- Explain that this exercise will demonstrate how it feels to have a confused mind.
- Ask participants to take out a piece of scrap paper and a pen, and place them on the table.
- Tell them to hold the mirror over their left shoulder and to locate the scrap of paper in their field of vision within the mirror.
- Ask them to draw a picture of a house by looking into the mirror rather than by looking directly at the paper.
- After they complete the exercise, ask for their reactions.

Alzheimer's disease is one of gradual deterioration. A person with the condition generally lives 8–10 years after diagnosis. It is important to realize that not everyone goes through the same stages in the same ways. Use Table 13 for general guidelines.

Table 13. Stages and characteristics of Alzheimer's disease

Stage 1	Stage 2	Stage 3
General		
• Appearance of stress • Exhausted, yet anxious	• Symptoms more severe • Increase in loss of intellect	• Close to terminal
Memory		
• Frequent need to check a clock and calendar • Forgets familiar names/words • Easily distracted • May not initiate familiar actions • Forgets answers/ repeats questions	• Loses important items • Hesitates with answers • Forgets directions • Slips in self-care • Obvious lapses in recent memory	• Recent and old memories very distorted
Orientation		
• Disorientation to time • May get lost • Confused with day and night • May forget meals	• Disorientation to person, place, and time	• Disorientation to time, place
Judgment		
• Difficulty making decisions • Spends money irresponsibly • May stop making decisions on the job	• May not observe precautions in traffic • May not be attentive to safety in own home	• Judgment usually absent
Learning		
• Difficulty concentrating • May struggle with familiar and easy tasks • Cannot make appropriate associations	• Cannot follow more than one- or two-step directions • Difficulty focusing on topic or subject	• Learning usually absent
Calculation		
• Problems in handling money • Frequent mistakes in bills and accounts • May lose ability to write	• Often cannot count change • Difficulty with arithmetic	• Calculation skills usually absent
Behavior		
• Person just not himself or herself	• Often does not express thoughts	• May be very unaware or indifferent

continued

Table 13. *continued*

Stage 1	Stage 2	Stage 3
• Loss of energy and enthusiasm • May lose interest in family affairs • May become accusative • May anger quickly • May not be as spontaneous or be slower to react	• May have extreme mood swings • May appear apathetic • May interpret words and places incorrectly	• May seem catatonic or coma-like • May be unable to communicate • May make only rare connections
Physical symptoms		
• May have frequent physical complaints with no evidence that something is wrong • May lose weight even though appetite is still good	• May have gait and movement problems • Restless • May have an overabundance of energy • May have some physical disabilities	• Very susceptible to infection • Incontinent (both bowel and bladder) • May still be ambulatory

Module 5

Caring for Confused Older Adults

Goal:

To increase participants' sensitivity to people who suffer from Alzheimer's disease or related conditions and to help participants master necessary skills

Objectives:

1. To demonstrate how to communicate with confused clients
2. To learn techniques for dealing with problem behaviors
3. To identify specific activities as interventions to help confused clients

Key Terms

Normalization activities: Those activities that provide the person with dementia with a sense of being a functional, productive person who is able to participate in life by doing the things she or he always enjoyed.

Task analysis: Breaking activities down into their smallest steps.

THE CAUSES OF DIFFICULT BEHAVIOR IN CONFUSED CLIENTS

People with Alzheimer's disease and related dementias often exhibit common symptoms, such as apathy, difficulty in concentration, confusion, and slow psychomotor responses. There is also a loss of problem-solving ability and abstract thinking. During the early stages of Alzheimer's disease, it is common for dementia and depression to occur together. People with early dementia are often aware of the changes and losses they are experiencing, for memory losses, judgment difficulties, and rapid mood changes can be severe enough to interfere with social activities.

Besides memory loss, dementia causes disorientation to time and place, inability to recognize people or remember names, visual perception problems, and language deficits. Dementia affects a person's ability to understand and to reason. It is important that the care provider understand the impact that these losses have on the client's ability to communicate effectively.

COMMON COMMUNICATION PROBLEMS

Confused clients have difficulty expressing thoughts in complete sentences. They may lose track of the point they are trying to convey and may easily get off the subject of their conversations. They often forget key words and names of objects and may experience the "tip of the tongue" phenomenon, which can be particularly frustrating. Their inability to express needs and emotions results in feelings of tremendous frustration. They may repeat words and phrases or invent words to fill the gaps. Words may be jumbled into a "word salad" that sounds like nonsense. (Figure 18 is a comprehensive list of common communication problems faced by clients who have dementia.)

Confused clients may not be able to grasp what is being said. The result of this misunderstanding is that they have a great deal of difficulty following instructions. If English is their second language, confused people often forget English and revert to their language of origin. The Guess My Line activity shows the difficulty of communication with confused clients.

GUESS MY LINE

- Have learners work in pairs.
- Have one person in each pair select a need to communicate. The person should not tell anyone what need has been chosen. The need should be communicated through rambling speech, "word salad," misused words, and so on.
- Allow 5 minutes for the other person to guess what is being said.
- For general discussion following the activity, ask the following question: How did it feel not to be understood? How did it feel to have to struggle to figure out what was being said?

- They are unable to express their thoughts in complete sentences.
- They lose track of their point while they are speaking.
- They get off the subject easily.
- They forget key words and names for objects.
- They cannot express their needs clearly.
- They cannot express their feelings clearly.
- They experience frustration when they are unable to speak clearly.
- They cannot understand what is being said.
- They forget English (if learned as a second language).
- They cannot follow commands (sequence of instructions).
- They experience a "tip of the tongue" feeling.
- They repeat words and phrases.
- They make up words to fill in missing phrases.
- They speak nonsense ("word salad").

Figure 18. Communication problems of people with dementia.

TECHNIQUES TO USE WITH PERSONS WHO HAVE DEMENTIA

When talking with someone who has dementia, it is best to use a normal tone of voice and to frequently call the person by name. It is better not to ask too many questions, but rather to make the questions into statements. "Let's go to the bathroom" is more effective than "Do you have to go to the bathroom?" (Figure 19 lists several techniques that can be used to communicate more effectively with clients suffering from dementia.)

- Speak in a normal tone of voice.
- Use the person's name frequently.
- Do not ask too many questions.
- Make questions into statements; for example, use "Let's go to the bathroom" instead of "Do you have to go to the bathroom?"
- Repeat statements or questions as often as necessary. Do not assume that you were understood the first time.
- Make negative statements into positive ones; for example, use "Come over here" instead of "Don't go out."
- Break directions and commands down into manageable steps.
- Wait until one step is completed before going to the next.
- Make and keep eye contact.
- Talk in a soothing, calm manner.

Figure 19. Techniques of communicating successfully with people with dementia.

Statements should be repeated as often as necessary because they may not be understood the first time. Negative statements should be made into positive ones. "Come over here" is better than "Don't go out."

When giving directions, the care provider should break down the commands into manageable steps and wait until one step is completed before going to the next step. The caregiver should make and keep eye contact with the client, while talking in a soothing and calm manner. The following activity gives the participants the chance to break down complicated tasks into simple, easily understood directions.

ROLE PLAY

- As a group, brainstorm simple, everyday tasks (e.g., having lunch, getting dressed for work, preparing dinner).
- Choose one of these activities and recreate it for a person with dementia.
- Ask for one volunteer to be the client. Try to choose someone who is not too shy—you want a little acting from the person in the role of the client. Instruct the volunteer to resist initial commands or to try to leave.
- Ask the others in the group to take turns giving each step in the process, one step at a time, until the activity is complete.

WHAT IS A BEHAVIOR PROBLEM?

Behavior is the way a person acts in a certain situation. In every society there are specific behaviors considered acceptable and others that are considered unacceptable. When a person behaves in an unacceptable way, it is said that he or she has a behavior problem.

Clients with dementia display many unacceptable behaviors that cause problems. "A problem for whom?" is the question that must be asked. These clients may behave in ways that make sense to them. The particular behavior in question may not be harmful to the client or to anyone else. Yet it is still considered problem behavior.

Some examples of behaviors exhibited by clients with dementia are wandering, pacing, repetitive motions, repetitive sounds, pounding/tapping on objects, putting things in the mouth, trying to leave, rummaging, hiding things, carrying objects around, getting restless during the evening, paranoia, agitation, anxiety, and sexual acting out.

The care provider should understand that people with dementia do not intentionally "misbehave." Their actions often occur because they misunderstand what is happening around them. It is the role of the worker to try to make the client as comfortable as possible by helping him or her make sense of their surroundings.

Causes and Triggers of Behavior Problems

Behavior problems may be caused by conditions that confused clients cannot understand. Hunger, too little or too much medication, being tired, needing to urinate, and pain or discomfort can trigger difficult behavior. Environmental stresses such as sensory overload, too much going on at once, and unfamiliar people or surroundings may also cause difficult reactions. The time of day may be another factor. It is common for clients with dementia to become agitated at sundown, sometimes called "sundowner syndrome." Frustration, depression, and the failure to do or say something can also trigger difficult behavior. (See Figure 20 for a comprehensive list of these causes.)

Most people can adapt to their environment and can adapt to changes, even abrupt ones, by altering their response. Those with dementia cannot adapt so readily, if at all. It is the responsibility of the care provider to reduce the environmental stresses that trigger problems. The relationship between clients and their environment is very complex, mostly because of the stress in the environment and the clients' inability to identify and meet their needs. As the diseases progress, clients lose their ability to cope. Their tolerance level for stress goes down.

These stresses directly affect behavior. Some stresses for the client can include the following:

- Not knowing where the bathroom is
- Being hungry, but not being able to relieve the hunger
- Wondering how to hold a fork
- Not understanding what people are saying

Case Studies

Mr. Jones probably can recognize the need to go to the bathroom and ask where it is. He can complete the task with the least assistance and remain relatively calm. His behavior is normal.

- Hunger
- Medication—too little or too much
- Tiredness, fatigue, lack of energy
- Environmental stresses—too hot or too cold
- Sensory overload
- Too much going on, too many activities happening near the person, too much noise, or just too many people attempting to interact at the same time
- Time of day
- Pain or discomfort that the client is unable to name or relieve
- The need to urinate
- Unfamiliar people or surroundings
- Frustration
- Depression
- Failure

Figure 20. Causes and triggers of behavior problems in people with dementia.

Mrs. Jefferson may recognize the need to go to the bathroom, but she cannot find the correct words to ask where it is. She begins to fidget and get up and down off her chair, and her eyes dart around the room. Her behavior is anxious, and she is losing the ability to deal with stress in her environment.

Mrs. Ross may feel a sensation but cannot connect it with "bathroom." She fidgets and wanders around the room, becoming even more uncomfortable. If she encounters some frustration at this point (a child running in front of her, for example), she may become angry or even attack the child. She has lost the ability to deal with stress.

DEALING WITH DIFFICULT BEHAVIOR

By adapting to their environment, people are also adapting to their own behavior. *Everyone is part of the environment. People can adapt themselves.* Because people suffering from dementia are unable to adapt to their environment, caregivers must be able to do the adapting for them. By adapting their own communication and attitudes, care providers can create an environment with less stress for the benefit of their clients.

Each client is affected differently by the dementing illness. Therefore, all clients will have their own stressors, whether it is the inability to find the bathroom or the inability to find or put on clothes. Each client will send different signals of discomfort: fidgeting, crying, increased wandering, or anxiety. The care provider needs to try to maintain the clients' dignity and encourage them to be as independent as possible. Caregivers need to take their cues from their clients by watching their reactions—this is the best way to determine what works. Then the workers can adapt their communication, attitudes, and environment according to what works best for their clients.

COMMON BEHAVIORS ASSOCIATED WITH DEMENTIA

Depression, Apathy, Withdrawal

Dementia clients often feel a sense of failure, feel left out, or have continuous obstacles to overcome in their environment. They may become sad or quiet and seem uninterested.

Wandering

Most professionals agree that there are two types of wandering. *Purposeful* wandering occurs when people are looking for something, someplace, or someone, or when they are wandering to get away from their immediate environment. If the wandering occurs because they have an abundance of energy or if this is simply how the disease has manifested itself, it is *not purposeful;* it is simply walking around. This instance is *not* a problem.

The following suggestions have proven helpful in working with wanderers as bedtime approaches:

- Try to create an atmosphere that encourages sleep. Try a warm bath at bedtime, a glass of warm milk, soft music, and night lights on in the bedroom.

- If the person gets up at night to go to the bathroom, leave the bathroom and bedroom doors open and the hall and bathroom lights on. Mark the bathroom and bedroom doors with reflecting tape so that these doors will stand out and the client can distinguish them.
- Surround the person with familiar objects and perhaps even special "holding" pillows or blankets. If the client awakens at night, she will recognize that she is in familiar surroundings.
- A person who awakens at night and is confused should be assured that he or she is in the right place, that the family is there, that everyone is safe, and that it is too early to be up. Often, this reassurance will be enough to get the client to go back to sleep.
- Exercise, when done regularly and adjusted to the client's capabilities and endurance level, provides a sedating effect. Walking is an excellent form of exercise.

Paranoia, Suspicion, Hallucinations

Clients sometimes accuse family members or others of taking their belongings. They may also see and hear things that are not really there. Dementia clients have a great deal of difficulty making sense out of their experience and environment. The disease has robbed them of their sense of well-being and ability to solve problems independently.

Restlessness and Sundowning

People with dementia seem to become more confused, restless, and insecure later in the day (toward sundown). They may also become more impulsive because they are responding to their own idea of reality.

Inappropriate Social or Sexual Behavior

Clients with dementia often begin to lose their inhibitions and sense of modesty. As the disease progresses, they have more difficulty setting their own limits. Care providers should, if possible, avoid making a "big deal" out of what is strange or inappropriate behavior. If Mrs. O'Toole were to walk out of the bathroom with no clothing on, it might be a natural reaction to say, "Oh, Mrs. O'Toole, where are your clothes?" and whisk her off to the bedroom. Pointing out mistakes and making a scene often embarrasses or humiliates clients, possibly leading to an anxious or agitated state. It is best to coax Mrs. O'Toole to a safe place, offer her some clothing, and help her.

Anxiety and Agitation

Many professionals now believe that anxiety and general agitation are not just a typical symptom of the disease but may be a reaction to stress.

Repeated Actions or Questions

Clients with dementia can become stuck in actions, such as continuously scooping their plate at mealtime or tapping their spoon on the plate. They also often ask the same questions repeatedly. Questions of the "I want to go home" nature are repeated frequently.

I Want to Go Home

Most people associate "home" with a feeling of comfort and security. Clients with dementia who do not remember where they are or who they are with are missing that feeling of security. They may say "I want to go home"—although they are really at home—because they do not feel secure.

HELPING CLIENTS WITH ACTIVITIES OF DAILY LIVING

Clients with dementia may need help with basic, everyday activities, such as grooming, dressing, feeding, bathing, brushing teeth, toileting, exercise, and leisure pursuit. There are two methods that are the keys to helping people with dementia do these activities. One is *repetition,* and the other is *breaking down the cues and commands.*

Task Analysis

When working with older clients, care providers often assume incorrectly that the clients can complete all of the steps involved in a task. Even what seems like the simplest of tasks may need to be broken down into more manageable steps. People suffering from dementia cannot figure out the sequence of steps in a task. They may make mistakes, become frustrated, or simply do nothing. This behavior is often misinterpreted as uncooperative. It is very important for caregivers to observe the clients with whom they are working and, if necessary, break down the steps.

TASK ANALYSIS

- Choose one specific activity of daily living, such as brushing teeth.
- Instruct participants to write down on a piece of paper the steps they take to brush their teeth.
- When they are done, ask them how many steps they have written.
- Ask someone with few steps to read her list. It may only include the following:

  Put toothpaste on the toothbrush.
  Brush teeth.
  Rinse mouth.
- Ask the other participants what is missing.
- On a chalkboard or flip chart, ask participants to help make a new list, including *every* step, among which should be, for example:

  Walk into the bathroom.
  Turn on the light.
  Pick up the toothpaste.
  Unscrew the cap, etc.

  Participants could mention more than 40 steps.
- This is the way clients with dementia must go about *everything* they do. The care provider's role is to make this process as trouble free as possible.

Cueing

Task analysis and cueing go hand in hand. Cueing means giving verbal or physical suggestions to help the individual with the steps of a task. There are four types of cueing. (*Note:* It is more important for care providers to remember what the ideas behind the cueing techniques are than to remember what the techniques are called.)

- **Verbal cues** use simple statements and emphasize key words: "Please *sit* down, Mr. Smith."
- **Visual cues** use props to show the client what the caregiver is talking about: "Mr. Smith, here is your chair. Please sit down."
- **Hand-over-hand cues** involve the care provider's hand being placed over the client's hand. The worker guides the client through the task while reinforcing the movements with verbal cues.
- **Physical cues** require care providers to use their bodies to guide the client's body through the steps. This is really a combination of all the cues. Use praise and encouragement in a dignified manner to let the clients know that they are successful: "Please sit here, Mr. Smith. That's good."

LEISURE ACTIVITIES FOR CLIENTS WITH DEMENTIA

"What should I do?" "Where do I go?" "Can I go home now?" Many difficult behaviors exhibited by people with dementia are a result of their inability to structure time and the frustration experienced as they attempt what used to be a simple task.

When care providers are aware of their clients' cognitive loss, they can work with their clients' behavior and interests to create positive experiences and opportunities for success. Rather than making clients fit into an activity, care providers can design activities for their clients. For example, an ex-golfer may still be able to hit a ball if it is in the right environment; an ex-secretary may still be able to sit at a typewriter and type, even if the words make no sense.

Everything people with dementia do, either for pleasure or out of necessity (eating, etc.), should be considered an activity. Clients go through the same difficult steps in brushing their teeth as they do in playing cards or knitting. The caregiver's approaches and interventions to both are the same. Although this chapter covers activities of daily living as a group and leisure activities as a group, both types of activities require the same structure.

THE VALUE OF LEISURE ACTIVITIES

Everyone likes to have fun and enjoy life. Dementia does not mean that a person cannot do so. However, it is necessary for care providers to structure activities so as not to cause the client to become confused and frustrated. Figure 21 emphasizes why leisure is so important for the client with dementia.

To get to know the client, the staff can interview the client (to the extent that is possible) and the family to learn what the client most likes to do. Remember that it is not always what the client is doing, but how he or she is doing it that is important. Both personal care activities and leisure activities

- To provide pleasurable passage of time
- To allow a person to pursue things that have always been of interest
- To distract a restless person
- To provide opportunities for exercise
- To increase opportunities for socialization
- To prevent behavior problems from developing
- To help a client feel like a worthwhile contributor to the world
- To encourage the highest level of independence that can be achieved
- To keep a client in touch with his or her past and present life and interests

Figure 21. Purposes of leisure activities.

can be adapted to allow the client the greatest possible chance for success. As difficult as it may be at times, caregivers must keep a positive attitude. Rather than thinking that a client "can't do that anymore," the care provider should think of ways to change the activity so that it can be successfully completed. Any accomplishment by the client, even a very small one like holding something while the care provider works on it, should be considered a success. If that task is the highest level task that the client can achieve, then that is an accomplishment.

REMINISCENCE AND NOSTALGIA

Reminiscence is an important part of everyone's life, especially older people. Care providers can draw out their clients and help them to re-experience events. Sometimes props can prompt someone's memory more than words can. Some items in the home that can be referred to for this purpose include the following:

- Old doll
- Scarf
- Toy fire engine
- Pictures of people
- Baby things
- Scrapbooks
- Bow tie
- Music box
- Baseball and glove
- Pictures of animals
- Scenery and travel pictures
- Old perfume bottle
- Tool box
- Old wedding picture
- Old postcards

TASK-ORIENTED ACTIVITIES

Certain tasks can give clients a feeling of usefulness and productivity. These tasks can be very effective with clients who are nervous or fidgety. Figure 22 lists activities that may be of interest to clients and can be fun for the care provider and the client to do together (Richman & Glantz, 1992).

Working with people with dementia requires the care provider to adapt to different circumstances. The caregiver can develop special techniques for working with confused clients. Understanding the causes of the condition and what the client is experiencing is important and helpful. When working with confused clients, the care provider can experience communication problems, behavioral problems, and problems with the activities of daily living. Knowing how to communicate with a confused person, using task analysis and cueing techniques, and creatively using leisure activities can make working with confused clients much easier. Working together is more rewarding for both the staff and the client.

Lower Level of Ability

1. Read a story
2. Start a game of cards
3. Review family photographs
4. Read poetry
5. Hold hands and share a special moment
6. Read a newspaper aloud
7. Exercise
8. Take a walk
9. Arrange a drawer
10. Clean a closet
11. Bring your clean socks and let the client or patient help sort and fold them
12. Put on makeup and give a manicure
13. Make an indoor garden
14. Take a car ride
15. Listen to some favorite records
16. Share a family recorded message
17. Make a scrapbook
18. Share a sack lunch or box dinner from home
19. Play horseshoes—indoors or outdoors
20. Make another client or patient smile
21. Join an activity program together
22. Study the Bible
23. Clip coupons
24. Paint a picture
25. Catalog shop
26. Reminisce
27. Have a spelling bee
28. Bring something from home to share
29. Sort buttons
30. Watch a balloon sail away
31. Take family pictures
32. Read your horoscopes
33. Re-pot a plant
34. Make a grocery list and discuss prices
35. Make a Christmas list
36. Decorate a small tree
37. Give a back rub
38. Set her hair, or let the client set yours
39. Make a no-bake recipe
40. Taste something new on the market—e.g., soda or candy
41. Play trivia
42. Practice buttoning a shirt, tying a shoe
43. Roll up skeins of yarn for future projects
44. Color a picture
45. Look through a magazine
46. Start a collection to work on together
47. Have a party
48. Make a birdhouse or small project to paint
49. Review the date, time, place

continued

Figure 22. 101 ways to use remaining capabilities of people with dementia. (Reprinted with permission from Rehabilitation Associates, Riverwoods, Illinois.)

Lower Level of Ability

50. Make a mobile for client's room
51. Bird or animal watch
52. Tear newspaper for garden mulch
53. Make a collage
54. Make ice cream
55. Pray together
56. Polish nails
57. Work on service project
58. Make some homemade lemonade
59. Pass out hugs
60. Have a tea party
61. Press flowers
62. Make holiday decorations
63. Have a picnic with all the trimmings
64. Think of 101 more things to do
65. Set a date—make plans for your next visit

Higher Level of Ability

66. Play cards
67. Work on a jigsaw puzzle
68. Work on a family tree
69. Play checkers
70. Write poetry
71. Plan the holiday meal
72. Do crossword puzzles
73. Talk about television show you have in common
74. Go for a walk
75. Make a craft project
76. Make family recipe book
77. Make phone call to someone you have not spoken with in a while
78. Polish shoes
79. Wrap a gift
80. Crochet together
81. Make party favors
82. Ask for some good old-fashioned advice
83. Sing
84. Watch and play television game show
85. What about those Bulls, Raiders, Bears, Sox, Angels?
86. Play cribbage or poker
87. Play lotto
88. Go over activity calendar and help make selections for the week
89. Make a list of things you like to do
90. Write a letter or card
91. Play tic-tac-toe
92. Quilt a lap blanket
93. Play bingo
94. Write an article for a newsletter
95. Travel and learn about a country through a book
96. Stencil some stationery
97. Give a book report
98. Share talent with group
99. Write your autobiography
100. Think of 101 more things to do
101. Set a date—make plans for an outing

Figure 22. *continued*.

Module 6

The Effect of Medication on Older Adults

Goal:

To educate the caregiver about medication abuse and misuse

Objectives:

1. To learn what constitutes medication abuse and misuse
2. To become aware of the factors that contribute to the abuse and misuse of prescription and over-the-counter medications
3. To know the signs and symptoms of potential medication mismanagement and abuse by older adults
4. To use appropriate intervention when dealing with this common problem

Key Terms:

Misuse: Improper use or treatment; to use incorrectly.
Noncompliance: Not taking the medications as prescribed or recommended by a physician or other health professional.
Polypharmacy: Prescription of many drugs at one time.
Psychotropic medications: Drugs that act on the mind; drugs that affect psychological function, behavior, or experience.

People are living longer than ever and, as a result, develop diseases and conditions they never would have experienced if they had died younger. In fact, people over 65 consume four times more health care products than do those under 65 (Simonson, 1994). People over 65 make up only 10% of the population but take 25% of the medications (Skeist, 1980).

MEDICATION AND OLDER ADULTS

Medication consumption by older adults is the rule, not the exception: Older people account for 30% of prescribed and 40%–50% of over-the-counter medications (Beizer, 1994). If older adults are healthy, they take an average of two prescription and one or two nonprescription drugs; if they reside in a nursing home, they average 5.15 routine medications and 3.23 more "as needed." Some people have as many as 30 medications lined up, prescribed by one or more physicians (Simonson, 1994).

The medications available today are very different from those of a few decades ago. Illnesses that were once fatal are now easily treated and controlled with medication. Among the most common conditions for which medications are prescribed are heart disease, hypertension, arthritis and rheumatism, diabetes, and mental or nervous conditions. Among the most commonly prescribed drugs are cardiovascular medications, tranquilizers, diuretics, and sedatives or hypnotics.

With medications so prevalent and so sophisticated, and with health maintenance organizations (HMOs) controlling doctors' time so stringently, the average visit to a doctor lasts less than 15 minutes and often focuses on medication (Skeist, 1980). Many doctors ignore the importance of diet, exercise, and relaxation to their patients' health. In addition, many people do not feel they have been helped by a doctor unless they leave the office with magic Latin words scratched onto little sheets of white paper (Skeist, 1980).

Older people do not, as a rule, abuse illegal drugs. They are rarely found in substance-abuse facilities, and they are underrepresented as overdose cases in emergency rooms. Yet more than 1.5 million people each year are hospitalized for problems caused by medication (Skeist, 1980); nearly one third of admissions of older adults to hospitals are associated with prescription drug-related problems, and up to half of nursing home admissions, according to a recent study, were associated with drug-related problems (Cooper, 1994). How is this possible?

Medication errors can occur at every step in the drug use process. These errors are made by both patients and professionals, the latter including the caregiver, the prescriber, the nurse or person administering the medication, and the pharmacist. The complexity of the new drug therapy, most of which was developed during the last 25 years, makes it almost a matter of life and death for clients to understand the medications they take, what these medications are for, what effects they should have and side effects they may have, their possible benefits, and their potential risks.

TRUE OR FALSE QUIZ

- Distribute the handout "Medication Use Quiz."
- Give learners 10–15 minutes to finish the quiz.
- Check the answers with the group and discuss implications.

☐ ☐ 1. Medication abuse means that the older adult does not care how he or she takes his or her medications. (False)
☐ ☐ 2. Not all medication abuse is addiction. (True)
☐ ☐ 3. Doctors always know everything about the medicines that they prescribe. (False)
☐ ☐ 4. If more than one doctor is involved with a patient, there is usually a good system for communication. (False)
☐ ☐ 5. More than a dozen people may be involved in a patient's drug therapy. (True)
☐ ☐ 6. Consumers need to learn how to inquire about what they should expect from drug therapy. (True)
☐ ☐ 7. The quality of drug therapy for older people is as clearly defined as for younger people. (False)
☐ ☐ 8. Health professionals, though often much younger than their older patients, understand how patients define quality of life. (False)
☐ ☐ 9. Large numbers of nursing home patients receive psychoactive drugs, even though they often do not have psychiatric diagnoses. (True)
☐ ☐ 10. Psychoactive drugs have been effective against most of the behavioral symptoms of nursing facility residents for whom the drugs are commonly prescribed. (False)
☐ ☐ 11. General Motors makes higher profits than do pharmaceutical companies. (False)
☐ ☐ 12. Some forms of noncompliance can be viewed as the patient's disagreement with the suggested drug therapy. (True)
☐ ☐ 13. The consequences of medication abuse are likely to be more serious in an older person. (True)
☐ ☐ 14. Up to one third of elderly admissions to hospitals are associated with drug-related problems. (True)
☐ ☐ 15. Drug companies spend more than $2.5 billion annually to advertise their products. (True)

Older people care greatly about their medications. For people suffering from one or more chronic complaints, medication may be the only thing that brings relief from pain or that they feel keeps them alive. Most older people see more than one doctor. Polypharmacy or "doctor hopping" results in the older person receiving prescriptions from several doctors without any of these doctors having knowledge of one another's prescriptions. A doctor might inadvertently prescribe a medication that results in negative side effects when taken with a drug prescribed by a different doctor, because he or she did not know about the medications already prescribed (see Table 14).

Some older people may not be happy with the prescription that they received. They might go to another doctor until they get what they believe is right. Or, if the pain or anxiety they feel is not immediately relieved with the prescribed dose, they might take an additional dose or give up on the medication altogether. Self-medication with the use of over-the-counter drugs can also cause problems. The dosage recommendations for adults for many over-the-counter drugs do not take into account the fact that an older body metabolizes the drugs more slowly than the body of a young or middle-aged adult. Warning notices are sometimes printed in such small letters as to be unreadable for many older people.

Unfortunately, older people are often passive when visiting their health

Table 14. Reasons for medication abuse and misuse

Problem	Effect
Polypharmacy or "doctor hopping"	Receiving prescriptions from several doctors *without* any of these doctors having knowledge of one another's prescriptions
Complicated medication regimens	Taking more than seven or eight medications
General poor communication with the doctor	Not fully understanding what the medicine is for, how it is to be taken, possible side effects, when it should be taken, and what to do if a dosage is missed
Memory impairment	Affects compliance, causing missing a dose or taking a double dose of medication
Sensory deficits	Vision or hearing problems leading to improper medication use—for example, difficulty reading small print on medication bottles, causing incorrect dosage
Self-medication	Because the pain or anxiety is not relieved with the prescribed dose, the client may take more
Mixing medications	Taking over-the-counter medications in addition to prescription medications, and neglecting to tell the doctor
Noncompliance with medication	Discontinuing medication because of unpleasant side effects or temporary relief; noncompliance can also be connected with feelings of shame or dependency about the medicine
Sharing medication or lay information	Taking someone else's medication *or* not taking own medication on someone else's advice

care providers. They were taught, and they believe, that the doctor is responsible for their health and should know what is wrong with them. The client must be willing to inform the care provider about all of his or her medical problems and symptoms of distress, including those "due to age" and those that "must be accepted," such as pain, constipation, fatigue, lethargy, and depression. Also, clients must inform each medical care provider about all the other medical providers that they are currently seeing. They must understand that they will not embarrass the provider or themselves by telling about other physician providers. The client should inform the health care provider about the following:

- Currently prescribed medications from all sources within the last 6 months.
- Medications used for past medical problems or once used for current diseases for which a different medication is now being employed.
- Results, both positive and negative, with past and present medications. Has noncompliance been a problem? Why?
- All allergies or intolerance to medications, including the nature of the reaction and what, if any, therapy was needed to treat the reaction.
- All nonprescription medications used routinely or occasionally (a good rule is any medication used in the last 6 months to 1 year), including a description of the conditions for which these agents were used.

Miscommunication with the doctor is a frequent problem. The older person may not fully understand what the medicine is for, how it is to be taken, when it should be taken, whether there are possible side effects, and what to do if a dosage is missed. Medication misuse and abuse are often accidental or a result of a lack of understanding about the medication and how to use it.

Complicated medication regimens—taking more than seven or eight medications—may be too confusing for the older person to keep straight. Some medications must be taken with food and others without. Some must be taken at exact time intervals; others give directions as vague as three times a day. For a person with some confusion or memory loss, remembering to take medications in the correct order and at the correct time is extremely difficult. The care provider can be helpful to the client when she has clear directions from the doctor, nurse, or family member regarding the reason for each medication and a definite schedule to follow. Figure 23 shows an example of a medication chart of the type used by caregivers to keep track of clients' medications.

Noncompliance with medication is a problem for everyone, not just for older people. In fact, you may find that many care providers also misuse medications. It is important for them to understand the correct use of medications for themselves and for older people if they are to be effective.

If there are unpleasant side effects, a client may discontinue using the drug. Conversely, a client who is feeling much better may discontinue the medication because it is perceived as no longer needed. This behavior is especially problematic for people taking psychotropic medications. These medicines must be taken for long periods of time to reach, and maintain, appropriate blood levels.

Another problematic but common behavior is taking someone else's medication. Relatives or friends may give the older person a pill from a prescription

Medication chart for:			Date:
Name of medication and dosage	Number of times per day	Time of day	Purpose
1.			
2.			
3.			
4.			
5.			
6.			
7.			
8.			

Figure 23. Sample of a chart used for tracking client medication regimen.

of theirs because it has done wonders for them. Or they may convince the client not to take prescribed medication because "it's not doing anything anyway."

Medication noncompliance is an issue that often confuses health care professionals. They do not understand why the person does not take his or her prescribed medicines. The care provider can give valuable information to the care team by reporting on the client's compliance or on observed side effects and behaviors. When a certain medicine does not agree with the individual, he or she may be better off without it or better off on another medicine. The caregiver can encourage the person to talk with his or her visiting nurse or doctor and not self-medicate.

Noncompliance can also be connected with feelings of shame about dependency on medicine. Often, people have the idea that taking medicine is not good or that doing so is bad for the body. In addition, different cultures have ways of healing that may not be the same as that found in the American medical system. The care provider may share the nontraditional views of some clients or feel strongly about medication in a way that is contradictory to the best interests of the client (or the health care provider!).

Many older people may be noncompliant for the simple reason that they cannot afford all the medication that has been prescribed. Instead of telling their doctor that money is a problem, they may do without, self-medicate with over-the-counter drugs, or pick and choose the ones they can afford.

Some people take medicine that is prescribed for regular use only when they have symptoms—for example, they might take high blood pressure medicine only when they have headaches or dizziness. It is important to be consistent in taking medication as prescribed. Skipping a dose makes high blood pressure worse. Many medications work only when a certain, consistent level of the chemical is reached and maintained in the bloodstream.

Although some older people are addicted to certain drugs, medication abuse is *not* limited to addiction. In fact, many abused medicines are not necessarily habit forming. Over-the-counter medicines, such as laxatives and cold formulas, can also be abused.

Doctors try to prescribe the most appropriate medicines, but they sometimes overlook allergies or other prior conditions. Encourage clients to keep medication cards in their purses or wallets, along with information about their allergies and other significant medical problems. It is critical for a person to have good communication with his or her doctor so that the client can mention how a prescribed medication affects him or her. For example, there is an increased risk of a serious drug reaction when a patient neglects to inform the doctor about the side effects she or he may be having.

Clients should know the following about each medication they use, whether it be prescription or over-the-counter: the name of the medication, what it is being used for, and the proper dose. In order to take the medication correctly, they will need to know the number of doses per day or frequency of administration, the best time to take the medicine, and the best way to take the medicine—for example, with meals. Some prescriptions must be taken until the medication is completed, others must be taken until symptoms are relieved, and others are ongoing. The older person should understand how long the medication needs to be used.

For people who are on more than one medication, it helps to know if the medication must be taken with other medications currently used, which medications can be taken together, and which medications must be administered separately from each other and how far apart they should be taken.

Not all medications are swallowed. Some medications are administered by special techniques or devices (e.g., inhalers, suppositories, nasal sprays). The care provider who will be reminding clients about medication must understand the preferred technique.

All medications have side effects. It is helpful for the caregiver to be alert to possible side effects of the most common medications. She can watch for telltale signs or ask the client if he or she had experienced anything unusual. If side effects seems to be occurring, the caregiver should notify her supervisor.

The older person may not understand the best way to store medication. Some need to be refrigerated, while others need to be kept in a cool, dry place. The bathroom may not be the best place! A nurse or pharmacist can help teach the older person the correct way to take care of medications.

TAKE YOUR MEDICINE!

The objectives of this activity are 1) to create empathy for the older person with some minimal disability who is trying to follow a complicated medication regimen, and 2) to graphically demonstrate some of the reasons for noncompliance. For this activity you will need the following materials: pieces of candy of varying sizes, medication cassettes, prescription bottles with child-resistant caps, others with easier caps, some "medication" in tubes, some eye drops, fingertip bandages, and adhesive tape.

Divide the class into small groups. If the group is small enough, ask the participants to put bandages on their fingertips and tape their knuckles to mimic the diminished sensitivity of the fingers of a person who has arthritis. An alternative is to have a few people volunteer to be the older person, with the others as observers or the caregiver.

Ask the participants to fill the medication cassettes, using the dosage directions on the pill bottles. Fill each bottle with a different-size candy. You may use the medication chart in the handout section or ask a nurse or pharmacist to give you sample medication regimens. Be sure to have some medications that must be taken with food and others that must be taken without food, some that must be taken every few hours, and others that must be taken twice a day.

Use the following questions for discussion:

- Did you understand the directions on the plan or on the bottles?
- How easy was it for you to open the containers and handle the "pills"?
- What do you think this is like for an older person with some memory loss or confusion?
- What do you think this feels like for a family member not familiar with medications?
- What are the legal limits of your job?
- How can you help?

When the activity is completed, participants can take their "medicine"!

SIGNS AND SYMPTOMS OF POTENTIAL MEDICATION ABUSE AND MISUSE

Older people may give the care provider clues as to how they are using their medications. These signs and symptoms may be either physical (i.e., what you can see) or verbal. A comment such as "I never like taking medicine" does not necessarily mean noncompliance, but it can be a clue in the presence of other factors.

The care provider can watch for both verbal and nonverbal signals that something is not quite right (see Figure 24). Signs and symptoms may include sleep changes (either sleeping more or sleeping less) and unusual dizziness.

A care provider may observe changes in the client that she may attribute to old age, pain from an illness, or suspected dementia. These include mood swings (unusually cheerful or unusually sad) and moving from one mood to the other; increased anxiety and irritability; and confusion, especially when there was none or little before. If a client who is generally good tempered becomes hostile or defensive, the care provider should report it to her supervisor.

Physical signs of possible problems include ataxia, trouble walking, loss of balance, and appetite changes. Clients who express problems with pain may not be using their medications correctly.

These symptoms can be caused by depression, medication problems, or other serious illnesses. As the eyes and ears of the medical team, it is crucial for the care provider to report these changes to the supervisor or nurse working with the client. Her job is to observe and report, not to interpret and diagnose.

- Sleep changes
- Unusual dizziness
- Mood swings
- Increased anxiety and irritability
- Confusion, especially when there was little or none before
- Ataxia (trouble in walking)
- Hostility, especially if this represents a radical change
- Loss of balance
- Defensive attitude
- Missed doctor's appointments
- Appetite changes
- Groggy or lethargic
- Difficulty managing pain

Figure 24. Signs and symptoms of potential medication abuse and misuse.

MISUSE OR NOT?

Ask participants to break into pairs or groups of three to discuss one of the following vignettes. Ask them to report back to the larger group the reasons for their decision, what problems could come from this person's action, and what they could do to help when working with this client. Allow 10 minutes of discussion for the small groups and a few minutes per group for reporting. An alternative would be to ask the small groups to role play the vignette.

Situation	Possible Response
Mrs. Smith forgot to take her heart medication yesterday, so she doubles the amount she takes today.	Encourage the client to ask the nurse or health professional what to do when a dose is missed.
Mr. Ramirez has severe heartburn, so he takes two extra-strength antacids without consulting his physician.	This is a medication that normally will not cause problems. However, Mr. Ramirez should report the symptom to his physician.
Mrs. Stein takes a laxative every day.	Laxatives should not be used daily. Mrs. Stein should be encouraged to regulate her bowels by using diet, increased fluids, and exercise.
Mr. Park's doctor has increased his dosage of insulin today. Mr. Park decides to continue on his old lower dose to save money.	Mr. Park should be encouraged to discuss his money concerns with his doctor or pharmacist. Perhaps there is a lower cost alternative to the prescribed drug, or a plan that assists in paying for medication.
Mrs. Glass feels that her arthritis medication is not strong enough, so she makes an appointment with her doctor to talk about increasing the dose.	This is the best way to work with a health care professional.
Mr. Zanitsky's wife is complaining that she feels depressed, so he shares his ulcer medication with her.	Medication should never be shared.
Mrs. Jackson notices that she breaks out in hives whenever she takes her pain medication. She has a doctor's appointment tomorrow and decides not to take the medication again until she sees her doctor.	A rash is a sign of an allergic reaction to medication. Not taking the pill is the correct thing to do.

Mr. McManus was prescribed 2 weeks' worth of antibiotics for a urinary tract infection. He feels better after 4 days and decides to stop taking the medication, saving the rest for the future.	Antibiotics are effective only if the entire course of treatment is followed.
When the care provider goes into Mrs. Farmingham's room to give her a bath, she notices a pill left in the medication cup. When she asks Mrs. Farmingham why she has not taken her pill, Mrs. Farmingham replies, "Oh, that's for my depression. But I feel so much stronger now. I don't have to take it."	Psychotropic drugs must reach a certain chemical level in the bloodstream—and stay at that level—to be effective.

WAYS TO PREVENT THE ABUSE OR MISUSE OF MEDICATION

One of the most important factors in being able to prevent medication problems is the relationship the care provider develops with the client. Building rapport and trust with a client is very important in creating a climate in which the client feels comfortable sharing feelings. When a good relationship is formed, a client may ask the worker to keep some things secret, especially if she is ashamed or is afraid of possible repercussions. Always let the client know that her confidentiality will be respected but that, in the best interest of her health and safety, information may be shared with her health care team (see Figure 25 for a full list of guidelines).

When medication misuse occurs as a result of lack of knowledge, the supervisor can involve other members of the health care team to educate the client on the right way to use the medication. Sometimes a client will more readily take directions from a care provider. The medical team or supervisor can educate the caregiver on the best way to use the medications. It is important to know the common abbreviations for medication use:

a.c.	before meals	O.D.	right eye
ad lib	freely, as desired	O.S.	left eye
b.i.d.	two times a day	os	mouth
c̄	with	p.c.	after meals
caps.	capsule	PO	by mouth
gtt	a drop	PR	by rectum
hr	hour	PRN	when required
h.s.	hour of sleep, bedtime	q	every
i	one	q.d.	every day
ii	two	q.h.	every hour

q.h.s.	every night	s̄s̄	one half
q.i.d.	four times a day	tab.	tablet
q.o.d.	every other day	t.i.d.	three times a day
s̄	without	ung.	ointment

Clients can be encouraged to keep records of their medication use (via calendar or medication cassette). Filling the cassette under the direction of the client or the nurse may become a part of the care provider's job. If an older person is having problems keeping track of a complicated medication regimen, ask the nurse to contact the physician for an easier one.

Help clients to correct sensory deficits, if possible. Make sure that they wear their glasses and use their hearing aids. Something as simple as not being able to see pills or hear directions can get in the way of using medication correctly. Use other techniques for managing stress, pain, and anxiety. Try relaxation techniques.

In the home setting the caregiver can keep a list of the names and dosages of all medications used. Review this list with the nurse or other care provider each time a new prescription or nonprescription medication is purchased. Ask if the new medication will cause any conflicts with the present therapy.

- The care provider is responsible for keeping an eye out for clues (actions, symptoms, or communication) and for reporting to a supervisor.
- Build rapport and trust with a client. This helps develop a relationship in which the provider can pick up verbal clues.
- Always let clients know that confidentiality will be respected but that, in the best interest of their health and safety, information will be shared with their health care team. This is particularly true if a client says, "I'll tell you this if you promise not to tell anyone."
- Your supervisor can involve other members of the health care team. A nurse and/or doctor can work with the client to educate the person on proper usage of medication. Sometimes misuse happens as a result of misunderstanding.
- If an older person is having problems keeping track of a complicated medication regimen, ask the nurse to contact the physician for an easier one.
- Be aware of other ways abuse and misuse can happen: taking someone else's medications, taking too much or too little medicine, stopping medicine on one's own, combining medications and alcohol.
- Look carefully at possible medication interaction. Notify a supervisor, a nurse, or the doctor involved, or encourage the client and family to do so.
- If possible, help clients correct sensory deficits—for example, make sure that they wear their glasses and hearing aids.

Figure 25. Medication abuse and misuse—how to help.

Have emergency numbers handy for contacting the medical provider, pharmacist, poison control office, and hospital, and be ready to use 911 in case of emergency. See if the community has any Vial for Life programs.

Encourage the client to discard all old medications that are outdated (have passed the expiration date on the label) or that are not presently used. If there are questions about old medications, the client can take the medications in a sack to a pharmacist, who can help sort out which ones should be discarded.

Encourage the client not to hoard and share old medications. A client should not refill old prescriptions ordered by previous health care providers without consulting the current provider.

If vials with safety closure caps are difficult to open, ask the pharmacist for lids that are easier to open, but keep in mind the potential danger of accidental poisoning should children gain access to the medications. If inhalers are difficult to use, an attachment called a "spacer" may help. If reading a label or drawing a syringe is difficult, purchase a magnifier or other helping device.

EFFECTIVE COMMUNICATION

- Each of the following statements is followed by three possible responses.
- Read the statement and then read the possible responses to the learners.
- Ask the learners to identify which response is correct, and why.

1. Statement: "My pain medicine is just not working. I took some an hour ago, and I still hurt! Bring me the bottle so I can take some more."
   Responses: a) "Here it is. It's too bad that this medicine isn't helping you much." b) "The directions on the bottle say once every 4 hours. Would you like me to rub your back or get you a cup of tea?" c) "Now you know I can't do that. The pain can't be all that bad."
2. Statement: "I just can't seem to sleep the whole night through. I keep waking up a few times a night."
   Responses: a) "That must make you feel awful. When did this start? Are you in pain?" b) "I know what you mean. I can't sleep much these days either." c) "Perhaps you could take one of your husband's sleeping pills."
3. Statement: "My sister thinks my doctor is wrong to give me these pills. She doesn't think they'll work—they didn't for her."
   Responses: a) "You should listen to your sister. She's had experience." b) "What medical school did she go to? Listen to your doctor?" c) "Do you feel that the medication is helpful? Why don't you take them as directed and talk to your doctor if you feel worried?"

A care provider who has an increased understanding and awareness of medication abuse and misuse will help maintain a healthier older population. Keep in mind that many admissions to hospitals and nursing homes are really due to medication problems, possibly undetected ones. Our common goal is to provide excellence in health care and to improve the quality of life as much as possible. It is our responsibility to be aware of risk factors related to medication abuse and misuse and to work with our clients and their families and physicians.

Module 7

Understanding and Recognizing Alcohol Abuse

Goal:

To alert the care provider to the issues and problems of alcohol abuse by older adults

Objectives:

1. To define alcohol abuse and alcoholism
2. To describe signs and symptoms associated with inappropriate alcohol use in older adults
3. To identify life situations that may predispose an older individual to alcoholism in later life
4. To develop an awareness of the special risks and problems associated with alcohol and aging
5. To identify appropriate interventions for caring for older adults who misuse alcohol
6. To recognize the barriers and stigmas that can interfere with identifying and treating this problem, including our own feelings, values, and beliefs about alcohol abuse in older people

Key Terms:

Alcoholism: A complex and chronic psychological and nutritional disorder associated with excessive and usually compulsive drinking.

Early-onset alcoholic: An alcoholic who begins drinking heavily in his or her youth.

Enabling: Actions by people in the alcoholic's life that help or allow the person to continue drinking.

Late-onset alcoholic: An alcoholic who begins drinking after the age of 40, usually in response to psychological or physical changes or losses.
Withdrawal symptoms: Physical problems that occur in response to withdrawal from alcohol. These symptoms can range from mild (tremors, sweating) to severe (hallucinations, seizures, and even death).

The first task, especially in dealing with such an emotionally laden topic as alcoholism, is to define the term. To understand alcoholism, it is important to remember that the alcoholic drinks excessively, compulsively, or both. Psychological and nutritional problems are often associated with alcoholism.

However, moderate, controlled alcohol use is not necessarily bad, nor does alcohol use by older people make them problem drinkers. For example, some people have a glass of wine a day and are healthy, well-adjusted individuals. In fact, some statistics suggest that moderate alcohol use may have some health benefits. Please emphasize the importance of looking at the *total* picture surrounding the client's alcohol use.

BELIEFS ABOUT ALCOHOL PROBLEMS

- Distribute the handout "Beliefs About Alcohol Problems."
- Allow 10 minutes for learners to answer the questions.
- Discuss answers. (The correct answer to each question is False.) Use the responses to discuss the myths surrounding alcoholism.
- Discuss the common beliefs about alcoholism being a disease or a character flaw. What leads to these beliefs? This is a sensitive topic, and care providers who look at some of their own issues connected with it can better care for their clients. Encourage discussion and sharing of values, beliefs, and (for those who are willing) experiences in their own lives or with clients.

Alternate Activity: Brainstorm

This quick exercise helps elicit myths and stereotypes about the older alcoholic. Ask learners what they think of when they hear that an older person is an alcoholic. Write participants' answers on a flip chart. By the end of this session, participants should have a better understanding of this issue.

ALCOHOL ABUSE AND OLDER ADULTS

Many people do not associate alcohol abuse or alcoholism with older adults. They think the problem affects teens or younger people only. The following facts about alcoholism will help shed some light on this serious problem for young and old alike (also see Figure 26). Although the rate of substance abuse is lowest among older adults, alcohol is the most abused substance. Drinking carries less of a stigma than do other types of drugs. It is also easier for the older person to acquire. A few drinks during the day are seen as normal or acceptable.

One study found the incidence of alcoholism in older adults to be surprisingly low. In the over-60 population, only about 5% of the population appeared to be alcoholic (Maddox, 1988). Other studies suggest that this figure may be low because chronic alcoholics tend not to live into old age, instead dying prematurely from diseases and conditions related to long-term alcohol abuse (Alexander & Duffy, 1988).

Drunk-driving arrests among older people increased 200% in the period between 1964 and 1982, a statistic that may be a consequence of the overwhelming growth of the older adult population over the past 30 years. One serious problem is that older drunk drivers are more likely than their younger counterparts to be released without punishment for their offenses, even though the older drunk driver is usually more dependent on alcohol than their younger counterpart and is predisposed to drive drunk again (Petersen, 1988).

Barriers to Treatment

A number of barriers, including negative societal attitudes, can interfere with identifying and treating alcohol abuse in older adults (see Figure 27).

Signs and symptoms of alcohol abuse in the older adult may go unrecognized because these symptoms mimic other problems related to aging. Slowed reaction time, confusion, and changes in sleeping habits could be a sign of depression, early dementia, or side effects of medication. Without looking for other signals, a person could say, "Oh, he's just getting old."

Society's negative image of alcoholism will often cause people to avoid talking about it. It is rare for a drinker to be confronted with his or her behav-

- Rates of alcoholism vary in the older adult.
- Generally, alcohol use tends to decrease with age.
- Although the rate of substance abuse is lower in older adults, alcohol is the most abused substance.
- Widowers have the highest rate of alcoholism; never-married women have the lowest rate.
- Alcohol use onset after age 65 is often connected with severe chronic illness, coping with a significant loss, and/or traumatic life experiences.
- From 500,000–2 million older Americans have some type of drinking problems.
- Of fatal motor vehicle accidents, 12% are related to alcohol abuse and involve persons 65 and older.

Figure 26. Facts about alcoholism.

- Signs and symptoms of alcohol abuse in the older adult may go unrecognized because these symptoms mimic other aging-related problems.
- The social stigma of alcoholism will often cause people to avoid talking about it.
- Feelings of helplessness occur on the part of us, the professionals: How should we handle this?
- It can be difficult to deal with the attitudes of the families of these clients.
- The feeling often arises on the part of both families and professionals that older people should be able to do as they like with the remainder of their life.
- Older people who abuse alcohol are more isolated.
- Lack of financial resources or lack of knowledge about available treatment choices keeps people from seeking help.
- Health professionals may have misconceptions about treatment of alcoholism in older individuals.
- Our own attitudes and beliefs, including a possible fear of addressing this issue, may keep us from helping the client.

Figure 27. Barriers to the treatment of alcohol abuse.

ior. It may be even harder to confront an older person in one's care. Although social drinking is an acceptable part of our society, alcoholism is not.

Care providers may feel helpless when faced with this problem. What do we do? How do we handle this? If we have not looked at our own general feelings about alcoholism, we may not be able to look realistically at alcoholism and older people. There are resources for the older person and suggestions on ways for the caregiver to discuss the problem with the client. However, the role of the care provider is to be the eyes and ears of the supervisor, nurse, or family. Care providers are in a key position to observe and report. Confrontation should take place only as a part of a carefully determined care plan.

Involving the client's family may be difficult. Family members may have ignored the problem or enabled or supported it (knowingly or unknowingly) for many years. We must be aware of our own feelings about the families of these older clients. Often the families themselves are in denial and cannot see the problem. Alternatively, they may try to shield the older relative because they feel uncomfortable labeling a grandfather or grandmother as an alcoholic. When this topic is broached with the families, health care providers sometimes meet with defensive anger or denial.

Another common attitude is that people of a certain age should do as they like with the remainder of their lives. You may hear staff members say, "Well, what does it matter? He's 90 years old. Who does it hurt?" If the older person is isolated, drinking may be seen as a consolation or a way to pass the time, not affecting anyone in any negative way. Older abusers of alcohol are more likely to be out of the work force, retired, at home, and widowed; younger alcoholics are easier to identify because of their higher visibility.

While alcohol rehabilitation programs are available in hospitals and medical centers, they can be expensive. A lack of financial resources may keep someone from seeking treatment. Also, the older person or his or her family may not know about available treatment choices. Treatment programs are often predominantly populated by younger people. The older alcoholic may feel out of place.

Last, and most important, our own attitudes and beliefs, including our fears of addressing this issue, may become barriers to treatment. No matter what our level of training, the subject of drinking is an emotional issue. On the one hand, we may value personal choice and the individual's right to make a decision about how he or she lives his or her own life—as long as it does not hurt another. On the other hand, we may believe that alcohol use or abuse is wrong. Another misconception is not realizing that substance abuse treatment can be successful, particularly for an older individual. The older alcoholic does not have to reach bottom before he or she can benefit from treatment.

The care provider is an employee. While she is at work, it is important that she works from the values held by the employer. Employer policy toward alcohol use by clients must be followed.

Early- and Late-Onset Alcoholism

There is a difference between early- and late-onset alcoholism. Often, different predisposing factors can contribute to the disease in both groups, as shown in Figure 28.

Early-onset alcoholics (or chronic alcoholics) are actually survivors of alcohol problems that began in their youth. They have been drinking throughout their life. As a result of the long-term chronic nature of their drinking, many early-onset alcoholics do not survive into their later years. Those who do often suffer from such chronic physical illnesses as gastrointestinal problems, liver

- Early-onset alcoholics or chronic alcoholics are actually survivors of alcohol problems that began in their youth.
- Late-onset alcoholics start drinking after the age of 40.
- Losses people experience as they age contribute to depression and can lead to increased alcohol use. These include death of a spouse, death or relocation of lifelong friends, retirement and/or loss of job status, financial insecurity, diminishing ability to drive, and deteriorating physical health.
- Late-onset alcoholism may be related to loneliness, boredom, and lack of purpose.
- Although loneliness and isolation can contribute to the problem of alcoholism, recent evidence suggests that problems with alcohol often develop in retirement communities where social drinking may be prevalent.
- Physical illness and depression related to a decline in physical health can lead to alcoholism.

Figure 28. Characteristics of an older abuser of alcohol.

disease, high blood pressure, heart disease, and malnutrition. They are also at increased risk for serious falls and accidents. Some long-term heavy drinkers may also suffer from Korsakoff's syndrome, a form of dementia directly related to long-term alcohol abuse.

Early-onset alcoholics may actually decrease their alcohol intake as they age because of their decreased ability to metabolize alcohol. They are at great risk for alcohol withdrawal symptoms, which can be life threatening.

Late-onset alcoholics start drinking after the age of 40. One third of all alcoholics over age 60 are late-onset alcoholics. Their alcoholism can be related to losses, severe anxiety, illness, and lifestyle changes. They usually suffer from fewer physical complications from alcohol abuse because they have been drinking for a shorter time. If treated early, late-onset alcoholics have an excellent chance for recovery.

Late-onset alcoholism is often called reactive alcoholism because it usually relates to external and situational factors. As people age, they experience many losses. Common losses include the death of a spouse and lifelong friends. If a person is accustomed to having a drink in the evening with his or her spouse or to go out socially and have a few drinks with friends, he or she may continue to drink alone when the spouse has died or the friends are no longer nearby. Although loneliness and isolation can contribute to the problem of alcoholism, recent evidence suggests that problems with alcohol often develop in retirement communities where social drinking may be prevalent.

Another common problem, particularly for older men, is retirement. If one's stature or sense of self has come from a job, retirement is a serious loss. Without a new role to take its place, a client may turn to drinking. For many people, retirement brings with it stress from a fear of loss of financial security. For a woman, being widowed can bring about a similar level of stress.

Men may see the deterioration of their driving skills as especially significant. Again, it strikes at their sense of who they are. Being unable to drive also makes a person more socially isolated, a frequent factor in depression.

Finally, poor physical health can be especially depressing to an older person. Alcohol originally may have been used to control pain, but the drinking then becomes more of an end in itself. Older individuals often self-medicate by combining over-the-counter drugs and alcohol.

Late-onset alcoholism may be related to loneliness, boredom, and lack of purpose, especially in retirees who never fully developed any leisure interests, or in people whose children or other close family members live far away.

Special Risks of Alcoholism for Older Adults

Age-related physical changes put the older alcoholic at special risk of alcohol-related problems (see Figure 29). Metabolic breakdown of alcohol in the body is less efficient in older people, resulting in higher alcohol blood levels than would be seen in a younger individual consuming the same amount of alcohol. What could be seen as moderate drinking for a younger person—say, two drinks a day—can be dangerous for an older person.

The reduced ability to metabolize alcohol affects many parts of the older person's body. The brain and central nervous system of an older individual are much more sensitive to alcohol, resulting in a very low tolerance. Older individuals who abuse alcohol are much more likely to develop gastrointestinal

- Age-related physical changes put the older alcoholic at special risk.
- Metabolic breakdown of alcohol in the body is less efficient in older adults, resulting in higher alcohol blood levels than would be seen in a younger individual consuming the same amount of alcohol.
- The brain and central nervous system of an older individual are much more sensitive to alcohol, resulting in a diminished tolerance. Alcohol depresses the central nervous system. It can cause depression or make an existing depression worse. Alcohol also accelerates the loss of brain cells.
- Older individuals who abuse alcohol are much more likely to develop gastrointestinal problems. Alcohol abuse increases the secretion of digestive enzymes, causing heartburn, ulcers, gastritis, and intestinal bleeding.
- Even small amounts of alcohol in an older person can decrease cardiac output and coronary circulation. Chronic drinking increases the risk of heart disease. Alcohol will make high blood pressure worse.
- Older people with preexisting conditions, such as lung disease and diabetes, can be especially at risk.
- Alcohol ingestion is especially serious for clients who take prescription medications. Medications can intensify the effects of alcohol, leading to rapid intoxication. Conversely, alcohol can decrease the effectiveness of the medication.
- Alcohol combined with sleeping pills can severely depress the central nervous system, leading to coma or death.
- An older alcoholic who stops drinking suddenly can face life-threatening consequences.

Figure 29. Special risk factors of alcoholism and older people.

problems, decreased cardiac output and coronary circulation, decreased respiratory effectiveness, and exacerbated diabetic conditions.

Alcohol ingestion is especially serious for older adults who take prescription medications. Alcohol combined with drugs such as digitalis, diuretics, insulin, antihypertensives, and tranquilizers can increase and intensify their side effects. Alcohol can even cause problems when combined with common over-the-counter drugs such as aspirin and ibuprofen. The combination can cause an increase in stomach irritation and bleeding.

An older alcoholic who stops drinking abruptly can face life-threatening consequences. Withdrawal symptoms can appear as early as 8–12 hours after the last drink is taken. Hangovers are mild withdrawal symptoms. Delirium tremens (DTs) are far more serious and may result in visual and auditory hallucinations, paranoia, extreme excitement, trembling, incoherence, and grand mal seizures. The DTs constitute a true medical emergency and need expert medical attention because they can lead to cardiac failure, shock, and even death.

Symptoms of Alcohol Abuse

Professional caregivers are in a key position to notice signs of alcohol abuse because of their frequent contact and relationship with their clients. However, it is often difficult to recognize alcohol abuse in an older person because the symptoms may be similar to other age-related problems (see Figure 30).

The care provider might suspect alcohol abuse in the client if abrupt changes in an individual's behavior occur, such as hostility, paranoia, disorientation, unsteady gait, slurred speech, and hand tremors. The key here is to notice a change. If the person was not originally hostile or paranoid and suddenly becomes so, the care provider should be alerted to look for other symptoms.

Frequent burns, falls, and abnormal bruising, especially at furniture height and on the backs of hands, are experienced by older alcoholics because of intoxication combined with declining motor skills.

Alcohol is an appetite suppressant. Decreased appetite with weight loss and pale, yellowish, or unhealthy-looking skin can be caused by poor nutrition.

Constant fatigue, frequent napping, and complaints of disturbed sleep may occur. Alcohol may originally relax a person and allow him or her to sleep as it is metabolized, but later it will stimulate the nervous system and cause sleep disturbances.

Alcohol use and depression frequently go hand in hand. A symptom of both is a deterioration in grooming and housekeeping. Clients may lose the motivation and the energy to keep up with their housekeeping or to keep themselves clean and neat.

Hangovers, blackouts, confusion, and forgetfulness are clear signs of alco-

- Abrupt changes in an individual's behavior
- Frequent accidents such as burns, falls, and abnormal bruising
- Weight loss and decreased appetite
- Pale, yellowish, or unhealthy-looking skin
- Frequent napping and complaints of disturbed sleep
- Constant fatigue
- Hangovers and blackouts
- Confusion
- Frequent headaches
- Deterioration in grooming and housekeeping
- Alcohol noted on breath
- Hiding liquor bottles

Figure 30. Signs of an alcohol problem.

hol abuse. Alcohol noted on breath and liquor bottles hidden in the living quarters leave little question as to alcohol use.

USE OR ABUSE?

Divide the class into small groups to discuss these cases. Using the "Recognizing an Alcohol Problem" checklists at the back of the book, determine whether each person has an alcohol problem.

Mrs. O'Connell is an 82-year-old widow who lives alone in a one-bedroom apartment in a retirement home. You have worked with her for a year. She has severe arthritis and walks with a rolling walker. She is very active at the retirement home and attends at least four activities a week. While bathing Mrs. O'Connell you notice a large bruise on her hip. When you ask her about it, she says she slipped on some water she'd spilled in the kitchen. Later, you notice an empty wine bottle in the trash.

Discussion questions: Had Mrs. O'Connell fallen before? Do you suspect that the fall was due to drinking? What other reasons could have caused her fall? Do you feel any further intervention is necessary? Why or why not?

Mr. Perez is a 76-year-old man who lives in a two-story home with his wife. Mr. Perez suffered a stroke 3 months ago, his second in a year. His left arm is paralyzed, and his left leg is very weak. He walks with a quad cane, and his left leg is braced. He needs standby assistance when he walks, for his balance is poor. He has a history of alcohol abuse, but he and his wife report that he stopped drinking after his first stroke. On your third visit you notice a strong smell of alcohol on his breath, but when you ask him if he has had a drink, he says no. You notice that his speech is slurred and that his balance is worse than usual.

Discussion questions: Does Mr. Perez's history lead you to believe he may be drinking again? Does he show signs of drinking? What are they? What should you do?

Mrs. Armstrong, a 68-year-old woman, lives with her younger sister, Mrs. Park, who has Alzheimer's disease. Mrs. Park moved into Mrs. Armstrong's apartment 6 months ago when it became unsafe for her to be alone in her own apartment. You have been working with Mrs. Park, providing personal care services twice a week, for 4 months. At first Mrs. Armstrong was pleasant to you when you came and would chat with you for a few minutes during each visit to express her appreciation for your help. For the past month, however, she has been distant. She looks tired and sometimes does not get dressed until after lunch. She has always been a heavy coffee drinker, and this week you noticed her pouring alcohol into her coffee when she did not know you could see her.

Discussion questions: Does Mrs. Armstrong have an alcohol problem? Do you have a responsibility to mention Mrs. Armstrong's drinking to your supervisor, even though Mrs. Park is your client? Does it seem that Mrs. Armstrong has always had an alcohol problem, or do you suppose this is a new behavior? Is Mrs. Armstrong's drinking a problem for her or for Mrs. Park? Why has Mrs. Armstrong started drinking heavily? What should you do?

Mr. Carpenter is a 72-year-old man who lives in a skilled nursing facility and has heart disease, Korsakoff's syndrome, and diabetes. He is ambulatory, though a bit unsteady in his gait, and able to take care of his personal needs. He has some short-term memory loss as a result of lifelong alcohol use. On occasion, Mr. Carpenter will leave the nursing home grounds and go to a bar. The last time he went out he was brought home by the police. He did not notice that a glass door was closed and tried to walk through it, resulting in a head injury. On another occasion, staff members noticed that Mr. Carpenter appeared drunk after a visit from a family member. A bottle of whiskey was found in his room.

Discussion questions: How does Mr. Carpenter's alcohol problem affect him and those around him? What is the role of the care provider? What is the role of the nursing home staff? How can Mr. Carpenter be helped?

Interventions with Late-Onset Alcoholics

A variety of treatment options exist, depending on the client's personality and other factors (see Figure 31). The care provider's primary responsibility is identifying and reporting symptoms to the supervisor. However, for the sake of increasing knowledge and understanding, general interventions/treatment options need to be understood.

Older individuals who abuse alcohol often feel very guilty and embarrassed about their problem. They grew up at a time when a terrible stigma was attached to alcoholism. Before it was recognized as a disease in the early 1950s, alcoholics were labeled as immoral, skid-row bums, and as weak-willed people.

People who are very important in the client's life—for example, family members, close friends, doctor, and religious advisors—should make clear and specific observations about problems caused by the drinking. There are differing opinions as to whether older alcoholics should attend Alcoholics Anonymous (AA) meetings with younger alcoholics. Some older alcoholics find that they cannot identify with the lifestyle of the younger people and are uncomfortable. However, others feel this mix of ages can be helpful, and many older individuals do not want to be in a group of only their peers.

- Build trust and rapport through day-to-day contact and conversation.
- Share concerns/suspicions with supervisor.
- Have intervention coordinated by a trained professional.
- Use a loving, gentle approach where concern is expressed and the client is encouraged to seek help.
- Encourage client to share feelings, especially those regarding illness and losses.
- Be nonjudgmental.
- Approach in the least intrusive manner.
- Promote alcoholic day-treatment centers.

Figure 31. Some interventions and treatments for alcohol abuse.

Another option for therapy is alcoholic day-treatment centers. These centers tend to be more sensitive to general issues of aging and special problems of older adults. They supply alcohol education, discuss general issues of health, and provide socialization.

The older adult may also benefit from attending programs at an area senior center or adult day care center. These centers provide social and recreational programs and may help in structuring the older person's day. Through developing social interaction and leisure-time interests, the person may become less depressed and isolated, lessening his or her emotional dependency on alcohol.

Antabuse is a medication sometimes prescribed by physicians for the treatment of alcohol abuse. It works as a deterrent by causing severe reactions such as nausea and vomiting when combined with alcohol. It is critical that the client taking Antabuse be monitored very carefully because it can have serious side effects, including severe vomiting, headache, loss of appetite, and loss of balance.

THE ROLE OF THE CARE PROVIDER

The care provider has the opportunity to build trust and rapport with clients through day-to-day contact and conversation. She can encourage clients to share some of their feelings, especially about illness or loss. When talking with older alcoholics, it is important to discuss their alcoholism in a nonjudgmental way. Words such as *drunk, drunkard,* or *alcoholic* should be avoided. When the older alcoholic is in denial (unwilling to admit to a drinking problem), he or she should be approached in the least intrusive manner.

If the care provider has any concerns about the client, she should share those concerns or suspicions with her supervisor or with another member of the care team. Intervention should be coordinated by a trained professional, not the caregiver. The confrontational approach, which is often used with younger alcoholics, is not appropriate for the older alcoholic. Instead, a loving, gentle approach is recommended, where concern is expressed and the client is encouraged to seek help.

Just as the symptoms of alcoholism can be mistaken for common age-related problems, the reverse can also occur. The stuttering gait of Parkinson's disease may be erroneously reported as the unsteady gait of the alcoholic. The acetone breath and coma of a diabetic in crisis may be seen as a drunken stupor. The forgetfulness, confusion, and poor judgment that are common in the early stages of Alzheimer's disease also may be mistaken for drunkenness.

The care provider must be a good observer and never make rash judgments in these situations, but must notify the supervisor of *any* unusual behavior or physical changes in the client.

Do not become too concerned because an older individual has an occasional glass of wine. Not everyone who drinks casually is an alcohol abuser. Clients should always consult with their physicians about alcohol use if they are on any medication, because the mix could be very dangerous. Care providers should understand that even though one or two drinks a day is normal for them, the same behavior may cause a problem for a client. They should know the effects alcohol has on the older body, on illnesses common in older people, and when mixed with medication.

Finally, caregivers should remember that sensitivity is very important in dealing with this problem. Most older adults are embarrassed and ashamed of their problems with alcohol. It is critical to deal with this issue in a caring, nonjudgmental way.

Module 8

Understanding and Recognizing Elder Abuse

Goal:

To give care providers the information they need to identify situations of possible abuse or neglect of their clients

Objectives:

1. To identify the types of elder abuse
2. To describe the characteristics of the victims and abusers
3. To learn the signs of elder abuse
4. To discuss interventions to use with the victim and with the abuser

Key Terms

Abuse: Mistreatment or improper treatment, including physical abuse, sexual abuse, emotional abuse, and confinement.
Neglect: Giving insufficient attention to a person who needs assistance, such as leaving the person unattended or uncared for. Includes both passive neglect and willful deprivation.
Financial exploitation: Misuse or improper withholding of another person's financial resources.
Dysfunctional: Impaired or abnormal.

At some time during their career, most care providers have known clients who were being abused or neglected. The caregiver may or may not be comfortable sharing this information with the supervisor. The information in this module is designed to enable care providers to identify situations in which abuse or neglect may be taking place. The next step is to report it to their supervisor. Clear reporting guidelines are helpful to care providers. Should they report suspected abuse or neglect to their supervisor or to the state elder-abuse hotline? (Note: The policy of the employer regarding situations of abuse or neglect must be known before this training can be conducted.)

Elder abuse is a complex issue that takes many forms. It can be defined simply as the physical, sexual, emotional, or financial exploitation of an older adult. The abuse can be either intentional or unintentional. Elder abuse usually happens in an older person's own home. Victims of abuse are generally isolated older people who are dependent on the abuser in some way. Most states have laws regarding elder abuse that include procedures for reporting suspected cases.

IS THIS ELDER ABUSE?

- Read aloud the following vignettes to illustrate the complexity of elder abuse from the viewpoint of the care provider.

Mrs. Alfano, 68, has had several strokes that have left her bedridden and unable to care for herself or even to tell what she needs. Ann, her granddaughter, and Ann's children live with her. Mrs. Alfano receives personal services from her care provider 6 days a week, and a nurse visits twice a week. Sometimes the nurses are not able to get in to see Mrs. Alfano because no one else is home. Mrs. Alfano's caregiver worries about Mrs. Alfano's treatment. She tells her supervisor that Mrs. Alfano is often left in her feces during the night and is not cleaned up until the morning. The granddaughter uses Mrs. Alfano's Social Security check and pension to pay the bills but did not pay the remaining balance for services from an earlier provider. Being responsible for someone who is totally dependent takes much time and patience. Ann gave up her job to stay at home and care for Mrs. Alfano. Caring for Mrs. Alfano is not easy, especially with children to raise as well. Ann is keeping her grandmother at home, where she feels that Mrs. Alfano wants to live. Is this really what Mrs. Alfano would choose for herself?

When Nancy's mother suffered a stroke, Nancy stepped in. It was a stressful job, caring for an older woman who could no longer control her bodily functions, and for Nancy the strain was too much. She began to abuse her mother: "I told her that her brain was like a sieve, that she couldn't remember. I'd say, 'If you don't stop messing up, we're going to stick you in a nursing home.'"

Nancy thought about suicide because the situation seemed so hopeless.

Mr. Cogliati is 78 years old and lives with his son, who is unemployed. The son is in need of money and cashes his father's Social Security checks for his own use.

Mrs. Patel, age 85, is retired and lives with her son and his large family. When she complains about the children bothering her, the son yells at her and sometimes strikes her.

Mrs. Cohen, age 70, has Alzheimer's disease, is incontinent, and needs constant supervision. Her daughter cannot cope with the situation. She ties her mother in a chair for several hours at a time.

- Have participants write down the things that concerned them about each scenario.
- Talk about their feelings regarding the cases they have heard and what they may have experienced in a similar situation.

TYPES OF ABUSE

In the United States in 1991 there were 227,000 reported cases of elder abuse. The National Center on Elder Abuse provided the following statistics on reported elder-abuse cases: neglect—45.2%, physical abuse—19.1%, financial/material exploitation—17.1%, psychological/emotional abuse—13.8%, sexual abuse—0.6%, all others—4.0% (Totara, 1993, see Figure 32). There are three main categories: abuse, neglect, and exploitation (see Table 15).

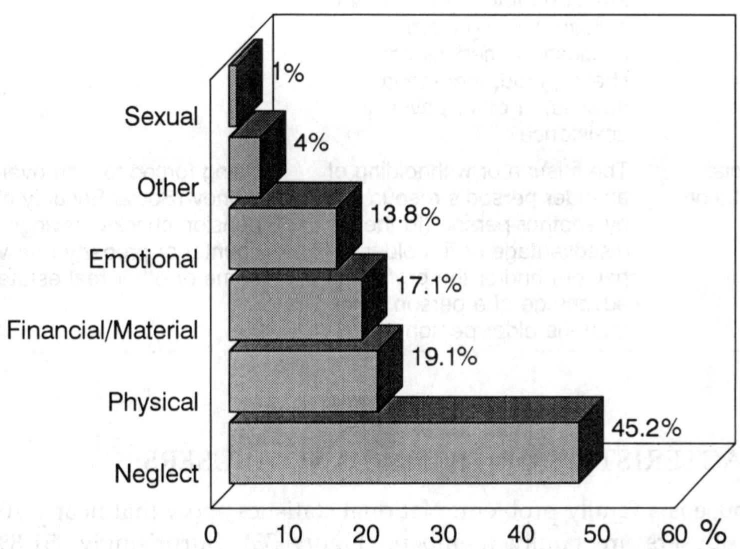

Figure 32. Types of elder abuse reported. (From Totara, 1993.)

Table 15. Types of abuse, neglect, and exploitation

Type	Definition	Example
Physical abuse	Inflicting physical pain or injury on an older person	Being handled roughly, slapped, or hit
Sexual abuse	Touching, fondling, or any other sexual activity with an older person when the older person is unable to understand, unwilling to consent, threatened, or physically forced to engage in sexual behavior	Being forced to be sexually intimate
Emotional abuse	Verbal assaults, humiliation, and threats of maltreatment, harrassment, or intimidation to compel the older person to engage in conduct from which he or she has a right to abstain or to refrain from conduct in which he or she has a right to engage	Being insulted, threatened, called names, or harassed
Confinement	Restraining or isolating an older person for other than medical reasons	Tying an older person to a bed or a chair to prevent him or her from wandering when he or she is not supervised
Passive neglect	Another person willfully withholding from or refusing to provide an eligible adult with the necessities of life, including, but not limited to, food, clothing, shelter, and medical care	Refusing to hire a cleaning service, neglecting to pay bills on time, and purchasing small amounts of food or poor-quality food
Willful deprivation	Willfully keeping from or denying older people, disabled people, or those in poor health the care they need; this can include denying them medication, medical care, shelter, food, therapeutic devices, or other physical assistance	Being denied food, clothing, shelter, medical care, or social contact
Financial exploitation	The misuse or withholding of an older person's resources by another person (to the disadvantage of the older person) and/or the profit or advantage of a person other than the older person	Being forced to sign over money (Social Security checks, pension checks, savings accounts) or property (the victim's home or other real estate)

CHARACTERISTICS OF VICTIMS AND ABUSERS

Elder abuse is a family problem. National statistics show that nearly 70% of the alleged abusers are family members (Figure 33). Surprisingly, 51.8% of the abusers are women and 42.5% are men (Figure 34). More than one half of the abusers are the victim's primary caretaker. The most prevalent abuser is a vic-

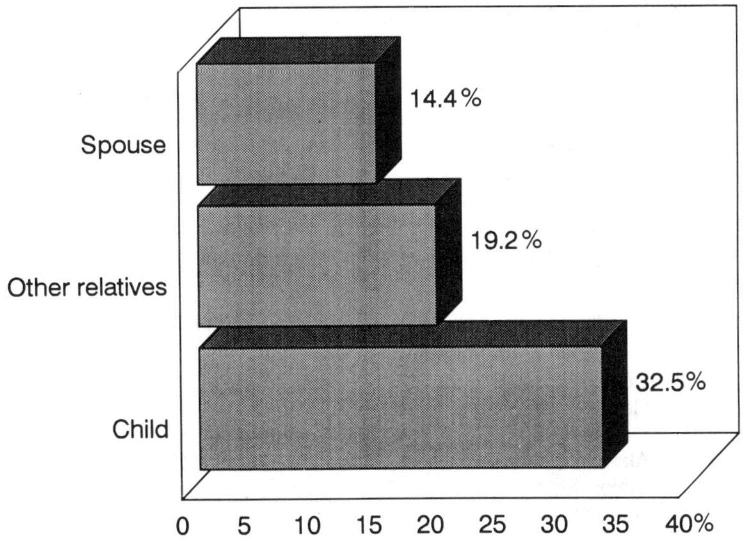

Figure 33. Abuser's relationship to the victim. (From Totara, 1993.)

tim's child (32.5%), followed by a spouse (14.4%), and other relatives (19.2%) (Totara, 1993; see Figure 33).

The abuser is most often a family member who lives with the victim. The abuser may lose control due to stress, may have alcohol or substance abuse problems, and may be frustrated and/or isolated. Abuse can be caused by economic or emotional dependence of either the victim or the abuser. The abuse may be accepted by the family as a normal way of life and not seen as a problem (see Table 16).

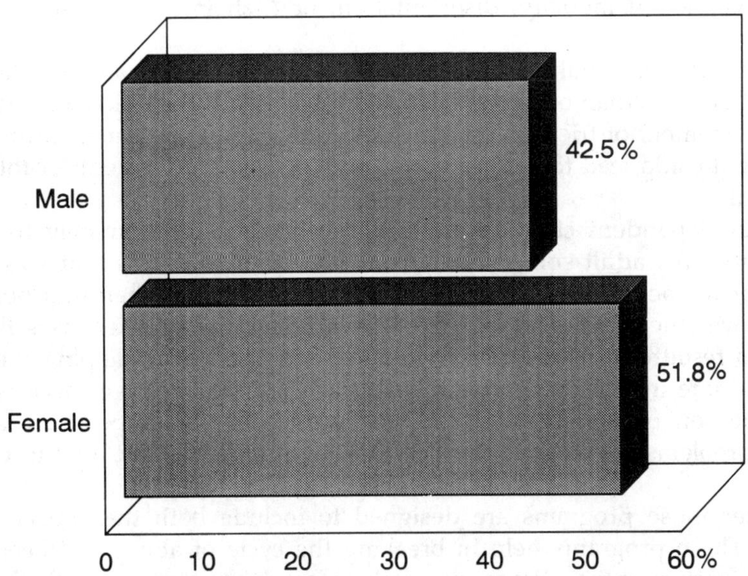

Figure 34. Percentage of abusive women versus abusive men. (From Totara, 1993.)

Table 16. Characteristics of the abuser and the victim

Abuser	
Factor	Frequency (%)
Substance abuser	24
Financially dependent	14
Functionally impaired	3
Mental illness	3
Other	13
None identified	52
Victim	
Factor	Frequency (%)
Functionally impaired	30
Nonambulatory	18
Hearing loss	15
Disoriented	14
Alzheimer's disease	13
Vision loss	13
Speech loss	11
Substance abuse	9
Other	14
None mentioned	24

Note: Percentage of domestic elder abuse cases/frequency of times reported, with the use of state aggregate data. Summary of the key findings of a national survey of state APS and aging agencies.

Data adapted from Totara, 1993.

Elder abuse is rarely a new problem in families; it usually involves a long-term abusive relationship. For it to be labeled elder abuse, the person being abused must be over the age of 60. Due to the larger number of older women than older men, 68% of the abuse victims are women; 32% are men (see Figure 35). Most of them have some type of impairment, functional problems, lack of mobility, disorientation, or Alzheimer's disease (see Figure 36).

The victim is usually dependent on the abuser for care and assistance and may suffer more than one type of abuse. It is difficult for a victim to admit that a family member or friend is an abuser. Or the client may fear reporting abuse, thinking it could lead to further harm, nursing home placement, or total abandonment.

Drug-dependent children often misuse their parents' money to support their habit. An adult son or daughter with a mental illness that was not detected or defined at an earlier age may well be abusive when in a position of power over the older person. The dysfunctional abuser often uses the older person's resources instead of generating his or her own. Helping the abuser become more independent may relieve the abuse. Supportive services can relieve the son or daughter's stress and reduce the older person's isolation. These problems are contributing factors in more than 25% of the cases reported.

Elder abuse programs are designed to include both the abuser and the victim. These programs help in breaking the cycle of abuse and keeping the family structure intact. Programs work to ease the stress on both the victim and the abuser.

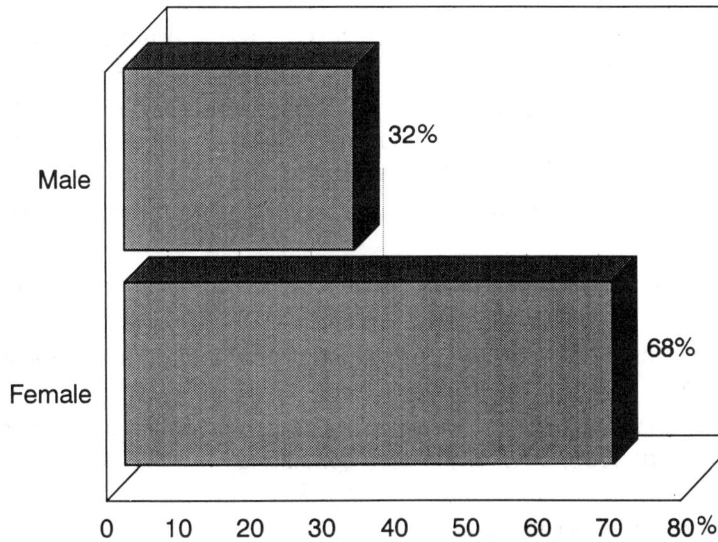

Figure 35. Percentage of abused women versus abused men. (From Totara, 1993.)

SIGNS OF PHYSICAL ABUSE

The care provider is uniquely able to watch for signs of physical abuse. (Figure 37 lists common signals.) When providing personal care, she is able to observe marks on a client's body. When taking care of the home, she is able to notice when items are missing or are needed and not provided. She may also observe abusive interactions among the people in the home.

Physical signs of abuse include bruises, welts, and skin discoloration. These may appear bilaterally on the upper arms, clustered on the trunk, or all

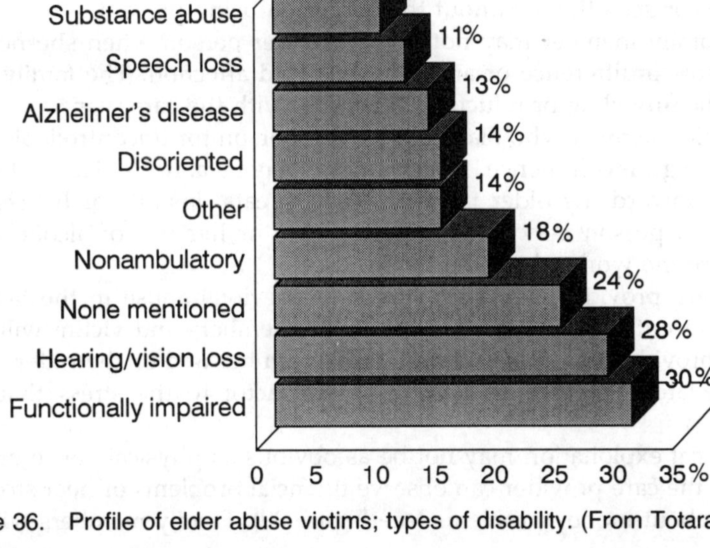

Figure 36. Profile of elder abuse victims; types of disability. (From Totara, 1993.)

- Bruises (sometimes shaped like an object), welts, bilateral discoloration on upper arms, clustered on the trunk, or all over body area
- Evidence of inadequate care (e.g., bedsores that have not been treated), soiled clothing and bed linens, lack of bandages or stitches when indicated, evidence of broken bones
- Poor skin hygiene, absence of hair, hemorrhaging (bruising) below the scalp
- Burns from cigarettes, acids, caustics; friction from ropes or other bindings
- Signs of confinement: client tied to furniture or bathroom fixtures, locked in a room
- Lack of necessary appliances (e.g., walker, cane, or bedside commode); lack of heat, food, or water; unsafe conditions

Figure 37. Signs of physical abuse.

over the body. There also may be evidence of inadequate care (e.g., bedsores that have not been treated), soiled clothing and bed linens, lack of bandages, lack of stitches when needed, or evidence of broken bones.

When bathing a client or helping her to dress, the care provider may observe poor skin hygiene, absence of hair, or hemorrhaging (bruising) below the scalp. Observable burns may be caused by cigarettes, acids, caustics, or friction from restraints.

Arriving for work, the caregiver may find the client confined, tied to furniture or bathroom fixtures, or locked in a room. She may also note the lack of necessary appliances (e.g., walker, cane, commode); the lack of heat, food, or water; and other unsafe conditions.

The care provider is also able to observe the interactions between people in the home (see Figure 38). Certain behaviors should alert the caregiver to look for abuse. For example, older people might not be allowed to speak for themselves or see others without their children being present.

The family member may not help the older person when she needs help or may show indifference or anger or withhold affection. The family member may also be unwilling or reluctant to comply with the care plan.

A family member who blames the older person for uncontrollable problem behaviors (e.g., incontinence, forgetfulness) may be abusive. He or she may be aggressive toward the older person, using threats, insults, or harassment. A signal that a person may be an abuser is his or her use of alcohol or other drugs while the worker is in the home.

The care provider may hear stories of previous abuse in the family. Accounts of recent incidents as told by family members and victim will conflict. The care provider will notice if the family member and/or the older person is socially isolated. Isolation is a contributing factor to the stress that triggers abuse.

Financial exploitation may not be as obvious as physical abuse or neglect. However, the care provider can observe financial problems or hear stories from the client about money problems (see Figure 39). Family members with access

- The older person may not be able to speak for herself or to see others without her children present.
- There are attitudes of indifference or anger toward the older person or an obvious absence of assistance.
- Family members blame the older person for problem behaviors (e.g., incontinence, forgetfulness).
- Aggressive behavior is shown toward the older person (e.g., threats, insults, or harassment).
- A previous history of abuse exists in the family (e.g., domestic violence, child abuse).
- Security or affection is withheld within the family.
- Problems with alcohol, drugs, or mental illness are observed.
- The family member and/or the older person is socially isolated.
- Conflicting accounts of incidents are offered by family, supporters, and victim.
- Family members display unwillingness or reluctance to comply with the care plan.

Figure 38. Typical abusive behaviors of family member or caregiver.

to an older person's money may seem to use the funds for themselves instead of the older person, resulting in unpaid bills or overdue rent. A care provider might see that the client does not have adequate food, clothing, or personal care items even when there seems to be enough money for these things. The older person may describe being grossly overcharged for rent or services, complain of being deceived, or claim to have had property or money stolen.

AVAILABLE INTERVENTIONS

Policies regarding suspected elder abuse should be clearly stated to care providers. They should include the person to whom the caregiver should report suspicions of abuse.

Care providers may be concerned that if they were to call an elder abuse hotline (if available), this action may be reported to their supervisor or to a

- A caregiver or family member with access to an older person's money appears to use the funds for his or her own purchases rather than for the older person, causing unpaid bills, overdue rent, etc.
- An older adult does not have adequate food, clothing, or personal care items when there appears to be enough money to provide them.
- An older person is grossly overcharged for rent or services.
- An older person complains of deception or theft of property or funds.

Figure 39. Indicators of financial exploitation.

client's family, perhaps to the abuser themselves. The caregiver should be reassured that the name of the caller who reports suspected abuse is not shared with the suspect. The approach of professionals who work with abusive families is to stress the desire to work with the client and family to resolve problems. Interventions are implemented depending on the older person's needs and wishes. The older person's right to self-determination is most important. If the older person is competent, his or her wishes direct the intervention.

Interventions may include the following:

- Chore/housekeeping services
- Nutrition services
- Adult day care
- Respite care for the caregiver
- Housing assistance
- Financial or legal assistance and protection, such as representative payee, direct deposit, trusts, order of protection, civil suit, and/or criminal charges
- Counseling referral for the victim and/or the abuser
- Guardianship proceedings and/or nursing home placement
- Emergency responses for housing, food, physical and/or mental health services

PROTECTING THE CARE PROVIDER

The discussion of elder abuse has focused on the older client as the victim of abuse, with the care provider observing the effects on the client. However, it is possible that the care provider will observe abuse or neglect as it takes place. On some occasions she may be caught up in a situation with a potential for violence, either to herself or to the older person. There are three things a worker can do to protect herself, and perhaps to protect her client: be alert for potential dangers, learn ways to defuse a potentially violent situation, and know when to leave (or not even to go in).

When the caregiver arrives at the home, she must be alert right from the start. Are there sounds of fighting through the door? Does the client or family member come to the door and refuse to let her in? If this person seems violent or shows signs of drug or alcohol use, the caregiver should not try to enter the home. Instead, she should report the situation to her supervisor.

Once in the home, the care provider must continue to stay alert. She should always plan a way out of the home. If there is a dog, she should ask to have it locked up while she is there. A dog cannot distinguish between physical touch that is helpful to its owner and touch that is harmful. The dog may attack the worker, believing it is protecting its owner. The care provider should not let people lock the door with a key. When working with the client, a bedroom or bathroom door should be partly open to hear what is happening in other parts of the home. If possible, the caregiver should position herself so that no one is between her and the door.

If the care provider observes situations in the home that increase her risk, she should leave. Some of these situations are when there is domestic violence taking place, the buying and selling of drugs, the presence of threatening and intoxicated people, or threats with weapons.

The care provider is often the one person outside the family who sees the victim of elder abuse. It is important that the caregiver be aware of the signs of elder abuse and understand the employer's policy on reporting suspected abuse.

IS THIS A RISKY SITUATION?

Discuss the following vignettes with the group. If the group is large, break into groups of three or four, giving one vignette to each group. Discussion questions include the following: How far should you go to protect your client? What should you do in this situation? How do these situations make you feel? How can you protect your client, and yourself, without resorting to physical violence? How would you calm a person who is very angry? Allow 10–15 minutes for discussion and a few minutes for each group to report back.

- You are making lunch for your client when her son, a known drug abuser, enters the apartment and begins demanding money from her. When she tells him she has no money, he threatens to hit her if she does not give him money.
- When you go to the Foley's apartment, Mrs. Foley refuses to let you inside. You can hear Mr. Foley in the background, and he's calling you to come inside and help him.
- Mr. Nelson's daughter, Jeanne, becomes angry at him for urinating on himself. She yells at him and slaps him. When you walk into the room to help Mr. Nelson, Jeanne tells you to get out of the room, saying, "I'll take care of him myself."

Module 9

Ethical Issues in Caring for Older Adults

Goal:

To increase care providers' awareness of the moral standards that they use in their work with older people

Objectives:

1. To define ethics and how they develop
2. To create a code of ethics for care providers
3. To discuss issues of confidentiality, job responsibility, elder abuse, substance abuse, sexuality, and money and gifts

Key Terms:

Ethics: The study of beliefs regarding obligations and moral duties.
Morals: Principles of right and wrong in behavior.
Value: A principle or quality that is thought to be desirable.

This unit examines situations that may arise in a client's home that will require a judgment call on the part of the care provider. By discussing tricky situations ahead of time, the caregiver will be acting on an articulated value. When supervisors share with care providers their beliefs of what is appropriate intervention, there is a greater likelihood of the worker responding in a way that the supervisor believes to be correct.

Training someone in ethics may be the supervisor's greatest challenge. Our ethics are the personal rules of conduct that tell us what is right and what is wrong. Training begins in childhood, when our parents set standards of right and wrong. To change one's ethics in adulthood is not an easy task. Yet it is often the personal rules of conduct held by care providers that will decide the quality and integrity of the care provided in the individual organization. This module was prepared with this thought in mind. The trainer can use all of the ethical situations identified, or choose those most relevant to the immediate situation.

Our behaviors stem from the values we hold. If we value independence, then we are more likely to do things *with* a client rather than *for* a client. If we value privacy, then we are more likely to keep quiet about our client's personal business. In times of stress, where a judgment call needs to be made, we frequently act on unspoken, internalized values. In home care, where the caregiver is on her own in the client's home, there are times where there is no clear right or wrong response. It is then that the care provider will take an action based on her own internalized value system.

DEVELOPING A CODE OF ETHICS

There are three steps to developing a personal code of ethics. The first is to recognize where our values come from, the second is to acknowledge what our values are, and the third is to realize the behavior that follows from a particular value.

ORIGINS OF ETHICS

- Have learners brainstorm where our ethics or moral standards come from.
- Write the answers on a flip chart or on the blackboard. Possible answers include family, church, friends, television, and school.
- Discuss responses with the learners.

Ethics Defined

Monsignor Charles Fahey wrote, "Each of us implicitly or explicitly, acts ethically; that is, we have established values which influence our behavior" (Fahey, 1983). What we value influences the way we act, with or without our conscious knowledge.

We learn many of our moral standards from our parents. They teach us right from wrong, both through their words and by example. If we have "internalized" what they have taught us, we carry these lessons around with us for the rest of our lives. They have become our moral standards, and we will probably pass these standards on to our children.

Our decision to work in this field is one example of how what we value influences what we do. People who value money over helping others will most likely choose a profession other than being a care provider. People who value working in a place where there are lots of other people to socialize with will probably not choose to work with a client at home. They may choose to work in a residential care setting, where there is interaction with other members of the staff. Those who value working independently while still being a part of a team helping older people are more likely to choose home care.

VALUES CLARIFICATION EXERCISE

- Distribute the handout "Values Clarification Exercise."
- Give the participants 10 minutes to answer the two questions.
- After the questions have been answered, invite participants to share their answers with one another.

THE ROLE OF THE CARE PROVIDER

The relationship the care provider forms with the client is key to the success of the care plan: "The helper's values, attitudes, and expectations hold particular significance in the formation of the relationship with patients or clients" (Sorensen, 1981). Having an empathic attitude toward one's clients sets the groundwork for a successful relationship. Empathy is different from sympathy. Sympathy is simply caring about people or feeling sorry for them. Empathy suggests an understanding of what is being felt without necessarily joining in the feeling. Having empathy allows the care provider to be understanding while maintaining a professional attitude and distance—to do tasks *with* a person instead of doing things *for* a person.

It is not necessary to walk in someone's shoes to understand what she is going through and to be sensitive to her feelings. One does not have to be the same age as their older client to be able to empathize. One does not have to be frail to be able to empathize with a frail person. Empathy for the client is important because one is less likely to pass judgment on the person's behaviors.

How each player in the relationship sees her role has an impact on the cooperation of the care team. Care providers may not realize that the client feels dependent upon them and how this feeling may affect their work: "Because of this dependency, clients do not view themselves as being in a position to go against the expectations of the helper . . . the client fears the power of others to withhold services and does not want to be considered a complainer or a troublemaker" (Sorensen, 1981). Those of us who value autonomy and independence will strive to develop a relationship that allows us to support the independence of the older person as much as possible while still completing the job tasks safely.

An important part of this process is to develop a personal code of ethics—our own commandments, our own mission statement—that helps us set our own standards for what is the right thing to do when our own personal judgment is called for. A code of ethics is important in any profession. Social workers, nurses, doctors, police officers, and most other human services professions have codes of behavior by which they expect participants to act. Professions have codes of ethics to protect the client, to protect the reputation of others within the profession, and to offer guidelines for behavior. Keeping in mind the principles of empathy for the client, the facility's mission statement, and the tasks of the job, we will now discuss some situations that commonly occur in the home and require a spur-of-the-moment judgment call on the part of the care providers.

CONFIDENTIALITY

Keeping information confidential means keeping it private or secret. Confidentiality allows clients to trust you with private information. The behaviors that follow from maintaining client confidentiality are not discussing your client or your client's problems with your other clients; not discussing your client and his or her problems with your family; not telling other family members what may have been said about them in anger, hurt, or disappointment; not discussing your clients with colleagues in a public place (e.g., on the bus, in a restaurant); and talking about clients only during staff meetings or in other official contexts.

When Should a Confidence Be Broken?

Clients may ask care providers to promise to keep certain information secret. There are situations in which one must reveal a secret. The caregiver should not promise to keep any information secret until it is clear that doing so will not affect the client's safety or the safety of others. If the promise has already been made, it will need to be broken. The following are a few situations in which the care provider should divulge secrets:

- If the client talks about suicide
- If the client talks about hurting someone else
- If physical, emotional, or financial abuse toward the client is suspected

The caregiver can report her observations in written records or report them to her supervisor. The caregiver may also be expected to report these changes to a designated family member.

CASE STUDIES

- Distribute the handouts "Confidentiality Vignette 1" and "Confidentiality Vignette 2."
- Give participants enough time to read each one before discussing the questions that follow.

CODE OF ETHICS

- Distribute the handout "Care Provider Code of Ethics."
- Ask learners to fill in the items on the handout as they are discussed during the session.
- Following the session, discuss learners' responses.
- Participants should keep the handout for future reference or post it in a place where they will see it often.

JOB RESPONSIBILITY

What do we mean by responsibility on the job? Clarity of job expectations is essential if care providers are to know what is expected of them. The work ethic of a supervisor and that of a caregiver may be two different things. Communication of specifics is important. For example, reliability is always valuable. Reliable to the supervisor means showing up at each clients' home exactly on time. Reliable to a care provider may mean being there within 15 minutes of the scheduled time.

Some examples of job responsibility that should be considered are the following:

- Report observations (physical, emotional) and changes to the supervisor
- Avoid being absent from work for reasons other than vacation, illness, extreme emergencies, or death in the family
- Be on time for work
- Do not gossip with other caregivers or clients
- Give sufficient notice before leaving

ELDER ABUSE

Care providers will occasionally witness abuse or neglect of their clients by family members. (Before discussing the ethical issues raised in witnessing possible abuse, teach Module 8 ["Understanding and Recognizing Elder Abuse"], which defines abuse, signs of possible abuse, and reporting procedures.) A care provider who witnesses mistreatment must decide if the situation merits reporting. Is it really abuse, or is this just the way the family interacts? Is her own position or safety at risk if she reports it? Does the client want her to tell the supervisor? Reporting possible abuse is one of those times where confidentiality may be broken. The safety of the client is the important consideration.

Just as with spanking a child, people will have different ideas of when discipline becomes abusive. A caregiver may feel that it is normal and acceptable to slap someone who is being stubborn or mean. The caregiver's background may teach that to fight back when struck is the right thing to do. When a client is verbally or physically abusive toward the care provider, she may feel she has the right to strike back. These values and behaviors may well conflict with a supervisor's goal of respecting clients and putting their safety above all else.

Talking about the experience of witnessing elder abuse is a way for caregivers to work through their own discomfort with a situation. When discussing case presentations, the trainer has the opportunity to model interventions and to more clearly define the abuse that has occurred. This also will provide the opportunity for care providers to look at their own behaviors that may have been abusive without them realizing this. The group can support the caregiver and suggest ways to handle the situation the next time it comes up.

Some guidelines that should be considered are the following:

- I will never hit a client, even if the client has hit me first.
- I will never swear at a client.
- I will never threaten a client.
- If I witness abuse of a client, I will report it to my supervisor.

SUBSTANCE ABUSE

Substance abuse is the mistreatment of the body by the use of mind-altering substances (alcohol or drugs). (Refer to Modules 7 and 8 for ways to identify when a risky situation occurs and when to report it to a supervisor.) As with elder abuse, substance abuse is an area in which the values of the supervisor and those of the caregiver may come into conflict. Therefore, it is important that care providers know the supervisor's stand on this issue. For example, a caregiver could be shopping for a client with diabetes and high blood pressure who asks her to pick up a six-pack of beer with the groceries. A care provider who drinks a six-pack a day will see nothing wrong with that request unless she understands the possible medication interactions and the employer's policy on purchasing alcohol for clients. The purchase of alcohol may be allowed unless a doctor says that alcohol is forbidden, but the policy should be discussed ahead of time.

Another example in which a care provider's behavior may preclude her noticing and reporting a problem is with the correct use of medication. Many of us do not completely follow doctor's orders when it comes to finishing a prescription or taking medication as directed. A worker who does not see the value of finishing a prescription may not encourage a client to follow the doctor's orders.

Some guidelines regarding medication and alcohol are the following:

- Never use drugs or alcohol on the job.
- Never purchase alcohol for a client who has a problem with alcohol abuse.
- Encourage clients to finish all medication as prescribed by their doctor.

SEXUALITY

One myth is that older people are not sexually active (see Figure 40). The fact is that unless the older person has an illness that interferes with sexual performance, he or she may continue to have relations. Older people also masturbate and live in "alternative" lifestyles—that is, have sex outside of marriage or are

Myth:	Older people do not have the ability to engage in sexual relations.
Fact:	While some illnesses may interfere with sexual performance, if the older person (as well as his or her partner) is reasonably healthy, sexual relations are possible into the 70s, 80s, and even 90s.
Myth:	Older people are not interested in sex.
Fact:	Overall, there is a decline in sexual interest with increasing age, but sexuality holds a place of great importance for most older persons.
Myth:	People who engaged in sex regularly when they were younger cannot continue this pattern into old age.
Fact:	Sexual patterns tend to persist throughout one's lifetime, and those who were sexually active in their younger years are the most active in their later years.
Myth:	Older people do not have alternative lifestyles; they are not homosexual, and they do not have sex outside of marriage.
Fact:	While they tend to be more "closeted" than their younger counterparts, older homosexuals certainly exist. There are also many older persons who engage in sexual relations with partners to whom they are not married.

Figure 40. Myths and facts regarding sexuality and older people.

homosexual. The care worker may be faced with a client who behaves in a sexual way that seems to them inappropriate. This is an area in which a care provider must show empathy and understanding and should remain nonjudgmental.

Care providers can be provided with the tools to use when faced with inappropriate sexual behavior directed toward them. It may happen that a client makes sexual advances, says things, or touches a caregiver in a way that makes her feel uncomfortable. The trainer and the group members can share stories and plan ways to respond to unwanted sexual behaviors.

Some guidelines regarding sexuality are the following:

- Gently, but firmly, rebuff sexual advances from a client.
- Consider the client's right to privacy and respect regarding sexual behavior.
- Regard sexual teasing as inappropriate behavior; a client may take seriously what we intend to be humorous.

SEXUALITY IN OLDER PEOPLE: A CASE STUDY

- Distribute the handout "Sexuality Vignette."
- Give participants sufficient time to read the vignette, and then discuss their reactions.

ACCEPTANCE OF MONEY AND GIFTS

A care provider has an unusual role in the care of the client. It may be tempting for the client to offer special gifts or extra money as a way to "ensure" good care. A caregiver who feels underpaid or believes that she has earned the extra money will be tempted to accept the gift (and not tell her supervisor).

Giving the care provider something may also be a way for the client to retain some feeling of control over the situation. Being the person doing the giving creates a feeling of power.

Accepting a gift may be risky. If the client is confused, she may believe the item or the money was stolen by the care provider. This is also a risk for the caregiver who is handling a client's cash for shopping. See Figure 41 for guidelines on accepting gifts and using cash.

ACCEPTANCE OF GIFTS: A CASE STUDY

- Distribute the handout "Money and Gifts Vignettes."
- Give participants enough time to read them, and then discuss their reactions.

Some guidelines on the issue of money and gifts are the following:

- Do not accept money or gifts from clients.
- Do not seek to manage a client's money in any way.
- Do not borrow money from clients.
- Do not ask to leave early and expect to be paid.

- Avoid asking for money or gifts from clients.
- Do not accept money or gifts from confused clients. Notify the family or the supervisor if you are offered money.
- Avoid managing the client's money in any way. Do not offer financial advice.
- Do not argue with clients about money. If the client refuses to pay, notify the family or the supervisor.
- Do not spend your own money on groceries, etc., unless you have worked out a plan for this with the family and social worker.
- Keep an accurate record on time sheets.
- Keep receipts of all items purchased for clients.
- Do not borrow money from clients.

Figure 41. Ethical behavior regarding the acceptance of money and gifts by caregivers.

Module 10

Dealing with Death and Dying

Goal:

To understand the natural stages of grief for the professional caregiver, for the client, and for the family

Objectives:

1. To discuss the importance of exploring the caregiver's personal attitudes and feelings about death and dying
2. To explain the characteristics of the grief process
3. To describe the many different ways people deal with the dying process
4. To demonstrate the way to give care based on recognition of the unique feelings, reactions, and needs of the terminally ill patient and his or her family
5. To express the need for all caregivers of older people to grieve

Key Terms

Acceptance: Agreement; admitting that something is true.
Bargaining: Reaching an agreement with another party that may be different from the agreement that both parties wanted in the first place.
Denial: Refusal to admit the truth or face reality.
False reassurance: Telling someone that everything will be better when you, in fact, know that it will not.
Isolation: Loneliness; the feeling of being set apart from others.

This module focuses on five major areas: 1) the importance of exploring and discussing one's personal attitudes and feelings about death and dying; 2) the characteristics of the grief process; 3) the many different ways people deal with the dying process; 4) the importance of giving care based on recognition of the unique feelings, reactions, and needs of the terminally ill patient and his or her family; and 5) the need of all caregivers to grieve.

Professional caregivers work with clients who are approaching the end of their lives. The task is to enhance the quality of life and the safety of people whose ability to take care of themselves has diminished or disappeared. The caregiver is constantly faced with end-of-life issues. How she has resolved feelings of grief from her own life experience has an impact on her work with the client.

When people grieve, they face the loss of a loved one, which in some ways is a diminishing of their own lives. The mourning process allows us to become whole. A new loss reminds us of previous losses. If the process of healing has not been completed, the new loss will affect a person even harder. For a professional caregiver, a client's death can bring up feelings of unresolved loss from her own life. The grief response will affect her work. A supervisor can support the care provider through the grief process, thus supporting them and enhancing their relationships with other clients.

The first step is for an employer to acknowledge the attachment that care providers have to clients and their feelings when a client dies. It is important for clients' deaths to be announced. Too often a care provider will hear of a client's death only when she receives her work schedule. This may be too late to attend a funeral or participate in mourning ceremonies with the family. It is important to afford workers the opportunity to put closure on their relationships in the way most comfortable for them.

Talk about normal grief and acknowledge the impact clients' deaths have on them. The following activity puts feelings into words, beginning a discussion about grief.

REMINISCING

- Explain that learners are going to spend some time getting to know one another.
- Ask learners to get up from their chairs and, without talking to each other, move around the room. As they walk around the room they are to silently choose a person they do not know and would like to meet. Allow about 60 seconds of milling around.
- Have participants choose a partner.
- Tell them, "With your partner, spend the next 10 minutes talking about your earliest memory of death—the death of anything or anyone."
- After 5 minutes, remind them to be sure to allow adequate time for both partners to share their experiences.
- After 10 minutes, reconvene the larger group and ask for volunteers to share their reactions

People experience a wide range of feelings when they lose someone or something. Terminally ill patients and their families will need to cope with their feelings of loss. A caregiver who understands and can identify her own reaction to loss will be better able to respond to the feelings expressed by dying clients and their family.

NORMAL GRIEF

Grief is a normal response to death and to any major loss. When someone or something important is lost, one needs to grieve. Each person's grief is unique. Yet there are some common reactions that people experience. Dr. Elisabeth Kubler-Ross, an expert in the field of death and dying, has found that terminally ill people and their families typically experience a sequence of reactions: denial, anger, bargaining, depression, and acceptance (Kubler-Ross, 1970). (See Table 17 for a summary of these stages.)

Denial and Isolation

The first reaction is to try to push it away. When people learn that they are terminally ill, they try to pretend that it is not happening. They do not want to think or talk about dying. Deep inside, there is the magical belief that if it is not thought about or talked about, it will not happen. Denial involves trying to avoid talking or thinking about the illness and the end of life. Terminally ill people feel isolated. They feel all alone, and they struggle with the thought that nobody else has to go through what they do. This is partly true because each person's experience with death and dying is unique to that person. It is normal for the terminally ill person and the family to struggle with feelings of isolation and denial. However, if there is enough time, it helps to be able to think and talk about the terminal illness and impending death.

Table 17. Stages of grief

Stage	Characteristics
Denial and isolation	The first reaction a person has is to try to push the knowledge away; it is normal for the terminally ill person and the family to struggle with feelings of isolation
Anger: "Why me?"	This is a very common question terminally ill people and their family members ask when they start to come to terms with the reality that the person is going to die
Bargaining	People often try to bargain by making promises to God or some higher power to allow them to live
Depression	It is normal for terminally ill people and their families to experience a sadness so deep that, at times, they may not be able to perform even the simplest tasks
Acceptance	The final step in the grieving process is acceptance; people may not need to talk a lot about all the thoughts and feelings they are experiencing, but when they talk about their illness and eventual death, there is a different feeling . . . a kind of a calm

Anger: "Why Me?"

This is the cry that is so often heard from people who are grieving the loss of someone or something important in their life. It is a very common question asked by the terminally ill and their family members, particularly when they start to come to terms with the reality of impending death. It is normal for the person to struggle with the question "Why me?," and to feel angry that he or she is dying while others are allowed to live. Anger and resentment often replace denial. People move back and forth, struggling with feelings of denial, isolation, anger, and resentment as they try to accept the reality of death.

Bargaining

People try to bargain by making promises to God or some higher power to allow them to live. This is a form of magical thinking that children use, but when under stress, we may think this way as adults. People try to gain strength from bargaining.

Depression

It is normal for terminally ill people and their families to experience a sadness so deep that, at times, they may not be able to perform even the simplest tasks. Dying is exhausting. Not only must the special needs of the dying person be met, but all the normal day-to-day needs of a family must also be met. On top of all this, family members need to cope with their anticipated future losses and review their past sorrow. Death is depressing enough just to talk about, let alone to live with.

Acceptance

The final step in the grieving process is acceptance. A person has accepted the loss when he or she is no longer angry or depressed. This is a sign that the mourning is over. Plans to die can now be made. In acceptance people may appear almost removed from what is happening. This is not denial or dissociation. They may not need to talk about all the thoughts and feelings they are experiencing. When they do talk about their illness and eventual death, there is a different feeling, a kind of calm. They have accepted the fact that they are dying.

Some dying people and their families may experience all these reactions; others may not. These reactions do not necessarily occur in sequence; more frequently, people move back and forth and may experience several reactions simultaneously.

These reactions occur with all of life's losses, not just dying. Unfortunately, everyone experiences losses. We grieve when we lose someone or something important to us, when we anticipate losing someone or something important to us, and even when we lose our hopes and dreams. To mourn life's losses is important. Yet, grief is hard work, and it is painful. Whatever the cause of our grief, healing takes time.

Some people have great difficulty mourning; they never completely grieve their losses. Unfinished grieving robs a person of energy. It numbs the feelings and diminishes the ability to experience love and joy. It sneaks up and pops out at inappropriate times, often when another loss occurs. Unfinished grief makes the new loss even harder to bear. Older people have experienced many losses in their lifetime. It is not unusual for an older person who is dying to think and talk about past losses and to need to review past sorrows.

Experiencing the loss of a loved one is never easy. However, many people go through the grieving process without knowing what is happening to them. Sometimes people who are grieving wonder, "Am I going crazy?" "Will the pain ever end?" The more understanding the caregiver has about what is involved in the grieving process, the better it can be handled. The care provider can be understanding and helpful with both others and herself.

RESPONSES TO DYING

- Assemble a number of photographs of ill and dying people from various sources.
- Instruct learners to gather around a display table on which you have placed the photographs.
- Have participants look over the photographs and choose a person to take care of. Advise the learners to not talk with each other while making their choice, to take their time choosing, and to look at each person carefully before they decide. Participants should choose one photograph.
- Instruct participants to return to their seats and, without talking to anyone, think about the following questions:
  - What type of care will this person need?
  - What will it be like caring for this person?
  - What were the reasons for your choice?

  Allow time for participants to think through the questions.
- Record the responses on a flip chart before the discussion.
- Discuss participants' responses.

The activity shows that each person perceives a potential patient or client differently. Occasionally, the same person may be selected or rejected, but for different reasons. Some will select a person for exactly the same reason others will reject him or her. Everyone perceives dying people according to his or her unique perception.

Realistically, the learners can base their selection only on the client's physical appearance. Some decide based on the person's likely personality—how verbal the person might be, and the anticipated difficulties in caring for the person.

People tend to form ideas about other people without being aware of doing so; they fill in the missing pieces of information to make decisions about dying patients and their families' needs. This "fill-in" information is based on personal experience, personal beliefs about death-related issues, and ideas about what a client might need in that situation.

Filling in information acts as a filter, screening out some things and selecting others. This filtering affects client care and also family care. However, "filtering" can harm the client, causing him or her painful feelings of isolation and alienation. It is a tragedy that some people must endure the pain that results from a caregiver's filtering. These people die feeling misunderstood and alone because the caregiver could not see or hear what they needed.

The job of a professional caregiver is to allow the client to go through all the stages of mourning. The caregiver cannot let her own fears and anxieties about a person's impending death keep her from sharing experiences, thoughts, and feelings. The dying person needs companionship and support.

Sometimes the caregiver's job is to help the client or family member identify and state their fears. Most discussions with dying people and their families focus on feelings. It is important for the care provider to discuss and explore her attitudes and feelings about death and dying. Her task with a dying client is listening with empathy and concern, not filtering.

THE SPECIAL NEEDS OF TERMINALLY ILL PEOPLE

Reluctance to discuss death is shared by many older people. *The dying person's preferences and his or her family members' preferences must be respected.* Some individuals prefer not to know about their condition. Some families choose not to tell the person that he or she is dying. However, most people who are dying know that something is going on, and they may be confused. Often, not telling people that they are dying is an expression of the stage of mourning known as denial. The primary reason for not telling is that thinking and talking about someone dying makes death real, and the reality of the impending loss of that person is very painful.

Husbands and wives may go to great lengths to avoid talking about the fact that the end is near. They may be frightened to talk to each other because of their unspoken fears over what will happen when the other one dies. A dying person may also avoid talking about dying to maintain the illusion of independence.

SPECIAL NEEDS OF TERMINALLY ILL PEOPLE AND THEIR FAMILIES

- Using a flip chart to record comments, ask participants to make a list of the special needs of terminally ill people and of their families.
- Distribute the handout "The Special Needs of Terminally Ill People."
- Give learners about 5 minutes to read the listed items.
- Discuss learner responses.
- Can participants think of anything to add to the list?

The caregiver's job is to be an active and involved listener who can keep her own attitudes, fears, and values to herself. Her role is to encourage the client in finding his or her own adjustment to death. The person who is dying may want to talk about the meaningful times in his or her life and to review the happy times of the past, or spend time talking with an impartial listener about the family and its future.

If the family is unable to talk about death, the client will turn to the care provider. He or she will look to the caregiver as someone who is comfortable having an open and frank discussion of death-related issues. In that way a care provider can help to put the client's practical affairs in order and help with issues of physical comfort.

The dying person has a right to control when and how physical care will be provided. As with any client, an explanation of what is being done during the giving of physical care should be provided. The client's need for privacy and dignity also should be respected.

The dying process may take a person out of his or her own home. The dying person may want to have personal items nearby: pictures of family members, sentimental objects, and other familiar articles. Along with comforting things, the client will want to have someone physically present to be there and care. The client will also want to participate in family rituals and customs as strength allows.

Many older people who are dying are not afraid of death. They are most often concerned about having to leave things unfinished, and they fear being ill and dependent on others for a long time before death comes.

TALKING WITH A DYING PERSON

Some people will seem to continue to deny death until the very end. When this occurs, people say such things as "I'll be better soon" or "If I could just get out of the hospital, I'd feel better." These statements show that the person cannot accept death. Take your cues from the client. If there is a resistance to talking about death-related issues, it may be helpful to ask this question: "Are you afraid of dying, or are you afraid of death?" When the client is ready to talk, he or she may initially react tearfully but then be open to talking about his or her concerns in great detail.

When the person is ready to talk, the caregiver should use factual terms and information and avoid using indirect terms or expressions, such as *going on, when your life is over, passed away, passed on,* or *end of life.* These terms tell the person that the care provider is unable to speak directly about death, so the client should not either. However, using indirect terms may be appropriate if that is accepted in the clients' culture. Sometimes the caregiver may be better able to talk with the person about concerns when family members are not around. Some family members cannot talk directly with their dying loved one because they are too overwhelmed by their own grief. However, when a person persists in changing the subject whenever the care provider tries to talk about death-related issues, the denial should be respected.

Sometimes neither the caregiver nor the client knows what to say. At those times, it is enough just be there and to hold the person's hand, brush the person's hair, make the person comfortable, or bring his or her favorite snack. That is all that is needed.

Religion is a very personal issue and is part of the adjustment to death. Some people find religion very helpful; others find it unhelpful. While particular religious beliefs favored by the person may not agree with the care provider's beliefs, this is not a time to argue. If the dying person or the family members ask the caregiver to pray or to read the Bible or other religious literature, she should do so if at all possible. However, the patient's beliefs must be considered. This is no time to impose personal beliefs on others.

Caring for the dying is always emotionally demanding. Not only do terminally ill people and their family members need to grieve, the care provider needs to grieve. She may need to seek and receive extra support from her supervisor or the health care team. This is normal! After all, care providers would not be doing the type of work they do if they had no feelings. There is no shame or embarrassment in asking for help; remember, everyone who grieves needs support—even professional caregivers. This is a good point in the discussion to remind learners of the "No One Is An Is-Land" exercise, which they completed in Module 3.

Care providers who are aware of their own responses to dying and death can discuss the way their own feelings and attitudes can "filter" this reaction to the client. Does a personal belief that death should not be talked about interfere when a person needs to talk about death? Do anxious and depressed feelings keep a caregiver from listening? Is talking about death difficult because it reminds the caregiver of her own past losses? Do care providers think that family members should not be upset with the dying person? These are but a few of the ideas, thoughts, beliefs, and needs that can get in the way of helping.

Module 11

Managing Caregiver Stress

Goal:

To improve the caregiver's stress management ability

Objectives:

1. To explain causes and results of stress
2. To identify coping strategies for dealing with stress
3. To review relaxation techniques

Key Terms

Burnout: Exhaustion of emotional or physical strength.
Coping: Dealing with and attempting to overcome problems and difficulties.
Stress: A physical, chemical, or emotional factor that causes bodily or mental tension.

Professional caregivers working with older adults have stressful jobs. They often work in isolation, seeing only their clients and their families. Their day-to-day stress may be compounded by their own family situations. This module examines what stress is, what causes it, how the body reacts to stress, the signs and symptoms of stress, and how to manage stress.

THE ELEMENTS OF STRESS

There are three elements involved in stress: the **stressor,** the **stress reaction,** and the **stress mediators.** The **stressor** is something that puts us on alert and ready to react. It may be a problem at work or at home, or it may be our own beliefs and expectations. **Stress reactions** are our physical and emotional responses to the stressor. **Stress mediators** are ways of managing that prevent us from experiencing a stress reaction when faced with a stressor.

Everyone experiences stress sometime in life. Some stress is important for a person's growth. Stress provides a challenge, stimulates alertness, and encourages creativity. Without at least some stress, life would be boring and frustrating. One might feel that strengths, talents, and skills were being wasted, and one could begin to question the very purpose of life.

Too much stress, however, is harmful. Called the "disease of the twentieth century," it is blamed for more illnesses than anything else known in modern life (Goliszek, 1987). Some diseases associated with chronic stress are coronary heart disease, hypertension, kidney disease, arteriosclerosis, chronic backache, gastritis, migraines, psoriasis, eczema, cold sores, shingles, hives, and ulcers (see Figure 42). The challenge is to find the delicate balance of just enough stress to stimulate life but not so much as to overwhelm it.

Stressors

The first step toward managing stress is identifying what causes stress in our own lives. Stressors include major life changes as well as the myriad of small, seemingly unimportant daily annoyances that can cause problems over time. Some examples of the latter are car problems, noisy neighbors, runs in stockings, too many parties at holiday time, rush-hour traffic, and leaky plumbing. Each person has his or her own unique list.

- Heart disease
- Hypertension
- Kidney disease
- Arteriosclerosis
- Chronic backache
- Gastritis
- Migraines
- Psoriasis
- Eczema
- Cold sores
- Shingles
- Hives
- Ulcers

Figure 42. Diseases that are induced by stress.

Stress Reactions

How does the body experience stress? Humans exhibit the same "fight or flight" response as other animals do. When a bird sees a predator, it responds immediately. If it feels that it is strong enough to win the battle, it stays to fight; if not, it flies away. This ability to react quickly enables it to survive.

The human stress reaction kicks into operation to help the body react to a stressor (see Figure 43). The numerous biological changes that occur during this process can be found in the figure. Stress reveals itself in many ways. A person's body, emotions, and behavior are all affected by stress. They provide clues to their response to stress. To manage stress effectively, it is important to recognize these signs (see Table 18) and identify the stressor(s) that triggered them.

Stress Mediators

People respond to the same stressor in different ways. One person may fall apart after a divorce, for example, while another may rally immediately. Stress mediators control the response to stress. They explain why some people can cope with stressful situations and others cannot. Not every stressor will result in a stress reaction. It all depends on the stress mediator:

- How we look at the stressor
- How we look at ourselves
- How we cope with the stressor
- What type of outside support is available to help us deal with the stressor
- Our physical and emotional condition

Perhaps the most important factor in handling stress is learning the difference between a minor irritation and a major problem. Not all battles need to turn into wars; even battles need to be chosen with care. This is a particularly important lesson to learn for the professional care provider, who frequently works with resistant or contentious clients. For her own peace of mind and to

- Heart beats faster
- Blood pressure rises
- Muscles tense to prepare for action
- Digestion stops
- Saliva dries up
- Sugars and fats are released into the bloodstream
- Breathing accelerates
- Blood-clotting mechanisms are activated
- Red blood cells increase
- Pupils dilate
- Senses are heightened
- Bowel and bladder muscles are weakened
- Perspiration increases
- Adrenaline and endomorphin are released into the bloodstream
- Endomorphin blocks pain, sometimes resulting in a feeling of euphoria

Figure 43. Changes in the human body that are induced by stress.

Table 18. Signs of stress

	Physical	
Headaches	Difficulty in swallowing	Facial or jaw pain
Dry mouth or throat	Difficulty in breathing	Tongue ulcers
Neck pain	Dizziness	Speech problems
Backaches	Muscle aches	Weakness
Constipation	Indigestion	Nausea or vomiting
Stomach pains	Diarrhea	Weight gain or loss
Rashes and hives	Chest pains	Heartburn
Heart palpitations	Frequent urination	Cold hands/feet
Excessive sweating	Insomnia	Excessive sleeping
Sexual problems	High blood pressure	Difficulty in sleeping
Swollen joints	Increased allergies	Chronic fatigue
Trembling	Accident proneness	Frequent colds or flu
Twitches		Menstrual irregularities
	Emotional	
Depression	Irritability	Difficulty in concentrating
Memory loss	Restlessness	Anxiety
Overexcitability	Nervousness	Nightmares
Impulsive behavior	Anger	Frustration
Neurotic behavior	Withdrawal	Feeling helpless
Indecisiveness	Feelings of panic	Disorientation
Suicidal tendencies	Confused	Frequent crying
Lack of interest in sex	Loss of control	
	Behavioral	
Pacing the floor	Increased alcohol consumption	Increased smoking
Gnashing or grinding teeth	Compulsive eating/ compulsive dieting	Nail biting
Foot or finger tapping	Nervous laughter	Sudden change in social habits
Hair pulling or twisting	Wrinkling forehead	Loss of interest in appearance
Increased medication use	Chronic tardiness	
Chronic procrastination		

avoid burnout, it is important for the caregiver to identify what triggers her stress with a client. Then she can learn her own way to manage the stress of working with a stressful client and give that person better care.

STRESS MANAGEMENT

A critical aspect of stress management is the avoidance of negative thinking. Negative people use the slogan "I can't do it" at every opportunity. Other people look at stressors in a positive way, considering them challenging and rewarding. Such people count blessings instead of misfortunes. Learning to look at life in a different, positive way gives one a feeling of accomplishment and strength when involved in a project. It allows people to look at change as exciting and possibly rewarding. People get a feeling of power when they take control of a situation. This can transform any stressful situation into a positive experience.

✸ MEASURING COPING STRATEGIES

- Distribute the handout "Ways To Cope with Stress."
- Instruct participants to read the explanation of each strategy. Allow about 10 minutes for completion.
- Review with learners their personal stories relating to the coping styles described in the handout.

The preceding activity is designed to help an individual identify the way she manages life's stress. Keep in mind that some stress is useful. The way people have developed to cope with stress is not necessarily harmful. Each method of coping is more useful at some times than at others. For example, when a stressor is too intense, it may be better for the person to withdraw for a while. As the situation changes, taking control may be necessary. The goal is to find a balance, using the best of each style.

The activity shows what can happen when a person uses one coping style to the exclusion of others. The handout describes steps an individual can take to modify her coping style to one that will work more to the individual's advantage.

How We Look at Ourselves

People must be realistic in their self-assessment and expectations. People are only human, not superhuman. All people have limitations and must accept them; every person must learn to set limits. It is perfectly all right to say, "I have had enough" or "No." These responses may be difficult for care providers, who, after all, come to work to help people. Many of them have a particularly hard time saying no to a client. They try to be superhuman, adding the stress of caregiving at work to the stress of their daily lives.

Perfectionist attitudes are not always healthy. Perfection is neither always possible nor always necessary. However, some people are in the habit of demanding it, and when it does not happen, they feel stress. Perfectionism also inhibits asking others for help, an important stress reducer. Perfectionists fear that helpers cannot do the job as well as they can.

Self-esteem—feeling good about oneself—is important. It is much better for people to be their own best friend than their worst enemy. If a person knows herself well enough to recognize when she is under stress, she can recognize the symptoms and try to change the situation.

✸ SELF-CARE INVENTORY

- We often look to others for compliments. It's nice to feel appreciated. However, these compliments may be few and far between. When they are given, they are often not what we had hoped for. To help yourself through difficult times, it is good to have a list of your strengths and assets that you can review.

- Distribute the handout "Your Best Qualities," and ask learners to write down five of their best qualities. Allow 3–5 minutes for this exercise.
- Tell the participants to take their list home and put it in a special place for future reference in time of need.

TIME MANAGEMENT

Stress often results from having too much to do in too little time. Learning to manage time reduces stress. If people take some time—no matter how little they have—to look at how they manage time, it will be time well spent. Learn to be realistic about time. How much can be accomplished within an allotted time? What is most important to do today, and what can wait until another day? List things to do, and set priorities (see Figure 44).

Leave time for emergencies and unexpected events. Consider delegating or asking for help. Asking for help does not mean you are weak or incompetent. It means you manage your time well and involve other people in tasks and problem solving. When working with an older client, keep in mind that your role is to "do with" the client, not always to "do for." Involving people in accomplishing tasks increases their self-esteem and strengthens their capabilities. Finally, schedule time to "stop and smell the flowers"; we often forget to schedule time to take care of ourselves.

Outside Support

When under stress, it is important to be able to turn to others for help. They can take on some of the work and responsibilities. They may offer additional support or resources. They may simply, but importantly, offer a listening ear.

- Take some time—no matter how little you have—to look at how you manage your time. It will be time well spent.
- Learn to be realistic about your time. How much can you actually accomplish within a certain period of time? What is most important to do, and what can wait for another day?
- Make a list of things to be accomplished. Leave time for emergencies and unexpected events.
- Set priorities.
- Consider delegating or asking for help. Asking for help does not mean you are weak or incompetent.
- Schedule time to "stop and smell the flowers." We often forget to schedule time to take care of ourselves.

Figure 44. Ways a caregiver can manage her time more efficiently.

Physical and Psychological Condition

Sometimes a person starts crying spontaneously over something that does not seem important or becomes angry for no apparent reason. The person may be in a state of weak mental or physical health and particularly sensitive to stressors.

There are ways to fortify oneself against stressors. Some of them are regular exercise, relaxation techniques, and good nutrition. Exercise may be as simple as walking regularly or as intense as working out at a gym.

Many relaxation techniques are available to professional caregivers, as shown in Figure 45. Ones that can be done quickly, easily, and when a person has only a few minutes include deep-breathing exercises, progressive relaxation, and meditation. These can be done when a worker has a few minutes alone, away from a troublesome client: in the bathroom, kitchen, or laundry room.

Deep-Breathing Exercises

Lie on the floor, with your head elevated slightly by a pillow. Your knees should be bent, with feet comfortably flat on the floor, about 8–12 inches apart. Place your left hand on your chest and right hand on your abdomen. Breathe in through your nose, taking in deep, even breaths to make your stomach rise. Your left hand should hardly move at all. Exhale through your mouth, whispering a sound like "aaaah." As you exhale, your jaw should be open slightly and your mouth relaxed. Repeat, taking deep slow breaths for at least 5–10 minutes. Breathing should be slow, regular, and relaxed.

Progressive Relaxation

Often you do not realize how tense your muscles become during a stressful situation. The following exercise will show you the contrast between muscle tension and relaxation.

- Sit quietly in a comfortable position.
- Close your eyes.
- Practice breathing (inhale through nose, expanding the stomach; exhale through nose or mouth, contract the stomach).
- Beginning with the right hand, tense muscles by making a tight fist, and concentrate on the tension.
- Hold for 3 seconds.
- Release the tension by uncurling your fingers and relaxing your hand. Concentrate on the relaxed state.
- Repeat tension-relaxation portion of the exercise.
- Continue the process using various muscle parts of the body.
- At various times during exercise, take a break, using the breathing exercise.
- Remember to tense and relax each muscle part twice.
- Concentrate on both the tension and relaxation.

continued

Figure 45. Relaxation techniques that can be used by professional caregivers to reduce stress.

Passive Relaxation

Repeat the steps above. Now try to relax every part of your body *without* first tensing your muscles.

Meditation and Imagery

Remove yourself from momentary stressors by visualizing a calm, peaceful scene. Focus your complete attention on a sound or image. This can reduce some of the physical effects of stress and help you feel calmer and more relaxed. Get in a comfortable position, close your eyes, and picture this:

> You are sitting on top of a grassy hill, overlooking the ocean. The sun is just beginning to set. It is comfortably warm as the sea breezes gently caress you. In the far distance, the water and horizon meet softly. The distinction of the two are blended into one mosaic. Notice how peaceful and content you feel. Carry your troubles out into the water. Release them and observe them float away with each passing wave. Stretch and exhale as you complete the exercise.

Stretching

An automatic physical response to stress is muscle tension. A simple, easy way to loosen tight muscles is to do stretching exercises. They take only a few minutes and can be done anywhere.

- Back stretch: While sitting, stretch forward, rest your body on your lap, and relax your head and neck. Hold for 1 minute, then press on your thighs to help yourself sit back up.
- Neck stretch: While standing or sitting, slowly rotate your head in a circle to the right without moving your shoulders. Then rotate to the left. Repeat five times on each side.
- Shoulder and arm stretch: Hold your hands together with fingers interlaced and stretch overhead with palms upward. Hold for 30 seconds, relax, and repeat five times.
- Passive back stretch: Lie on the floor with your legs on a chair. Relax, pressing your lower back onto the floor. Rest in this position for several minutes.
- Upper body stretch: With your feet a shoulder's width apart, reach overhead and stretch to the side. Try not to move your hips. Hold for 30 seconds; then switch sides.

Figure 45. *continued*

Good nutrition gives the body the strength it needs to handle the effects of stress. A well-balanced diet provides vitamins, minerals, carbohydrates, proteins, and some fats. It is important to eat a variety of foods from each of the four major food groups.

Caffeine content is an important consideration. Foods high in caffeine, such as coffee, tea, and chocolate, tend to make a person more anxious and nervous than usual. This is because caffeine is a stimulant.

STRESSFUL SCENARIOS

Care providers are often faced with stressful situations when they are working alone in a home or a client's room. It is useful to discuss with the care staff what could happen with a client. When faced with the stressor, the care provider will then be able to think of useful tips. She can respond in a way that is in the best interest of the client and herself.

TENSE SITUATIONS

- Distribute the handout "Stress in Caring for Older People: Vignettes."
- Ask participants to select the most appropriate answer for each scenario.
- Discuss learner responses.

Module 1

Facts About Older Americans

- In 1992 there were more than 30 million people over 65. By the year 2000, there will be more than 34 million.
- One out of every eight people is 65 years of age or older.
- About 5%, or a little over 1 million, of people over 65 years old live in institutions of one kind or another.
- About 9 million older people live alone or with nonrelatives.
- There are 150 older women for every 100 older men.
- Most older men are married. Most older women are widowed. There are five times as many widows as widowers, and half of all women in this group are widows.
- Of all older adults, 86% suffer from one or more chronic health conditions of varying degrees of severity.
- Of all people over 65 years old, 23% are limited in their activities of daily living due to chronic health conditions.
- Of people over age 85, 49% have difficulty with the activities of daily living.
- Among people over 65, 41% of women live alone, as compared to 16% of the men.
- The majority of people over age 65 who live alone will eventually be institutionalized.
- The fastest-growing age group of the population of the United States is adults over 85 years.
- In 1980 over 2.5 million people, or 10% of the population 65 and older, were nonwhite. It is expected that by 2050, 15% will be nonwhite, and by 2050, 20%.
- People over 65 go to doctors an average of eight times a year, compared to five times a year for people under 65.
- People over 65 are hospitalized twice as often as people under 65, their hospital visits average 50% longer, and they use twice as many prescription drugs.

Adapted from National Center for Health Statistics.

Module 1

Attitudes Toward Aging

1. What makes a person seem young?
2. What makes a person seem old?
3. Think about two people who know who are in their 70s. One seems young, and one seems old. Why?
4. What do older people have now that they did not have when they were younger?
5. What did older people have when they were younger that they do not have now?
6. Imagine yourself as an older person. What will you do for enjoyment? With whom will you spend your time? Where will you live?
7. What do you fear most about aging?
8. What do you look forward to in your older years?
9. How do your attitudes about aging affect your work with older people?

Adapted from *Older Persons and Service Providers: An Instructor's Training Guide*, by Gloria Sorensen, 1981. New York: Human Sciences Press, Inc.

Module 1

What's Your Aging I.Q.?

		True	False
1.	Baby boomers are the fastest growing segment of the population.	☐	☐
2.	Families don't bother with their older relatives.	☐	☐
3.	All people become confused or forgetful if they live long enough.	☐	☐
4.	You can be too old to exercise.	☐	☐
5.	Heart disease is a much bigger problem for older men than for older women.	☐	☐
6.	The older you get, the less you sleep.	☐	☐
7.	People should watch their weight as they age.	☐	☐
8.	Most older people are depressed. Why shouldn't they be?	☐	☐
9.	There's no point in screening older people for cancer because they can't be treated.	☐	☐
10.	Older people take more medications than younger people do.	☐	☐
11.	People begin to lose interest in sex around age 55.	☐	☐
12.	If your parents had Alzheimer's disease, you will inevitably get it.	☐	☐
13.	Diet and exercise reduce the risk of osteoporosis.	☐	☐
14.	As your body changes with age, so does your personality.	☐	☐
15.	Older people might as well accept urinary accidents as a fact of life.	☐	☐
16.	Suicide is mainly a problem for teenagers.	☐	☐
17.	Falls and injuries "just happen" to older people.	☐	☐
18.	All people get cataracts.	☐	☐

19. Extremes of heat and cold can be especially dangerous for older people. ☐ ☐
20. "You can't teach an old dog new tricks." ☐ ☐

From National Institute on Aging, 1991 Publication HP10, Washington, D.C.

Module 1

Sensory Dysfunction Exercise

Blindfolded and with guidance of a partner:

1. Go to washroom and use it.
2. Walk around room, through narrow space, through a doorway.
3. Ascend and descend stairs.
4. Walk to table and chairs, sit down.
5. Cut five pieces of yarn measured between tape.

With right arm and leg totally "paralyzed," sitting in a wheelchair:

1. Put on and remove a shirt, buttoning and unbuttoning the buttons.
2. File your nails.
3. Wheel your wheelchair 10 feet: forward, backward, right, and left.

First with smeared glasses and gloves, then with taped fingers:

1. Go to your purse or pocket, take out four coins, and identify them.
2. Open and close a safety pin and a bottle.
3. Button and unbutton four buttons on the shirt.

With blocked visual-field glasses:

1. Comb your hair, or put on lipstick.
2. Write your name.

Adapted from Richman & Glantz, 1992b.

Module 2

The Communication Process

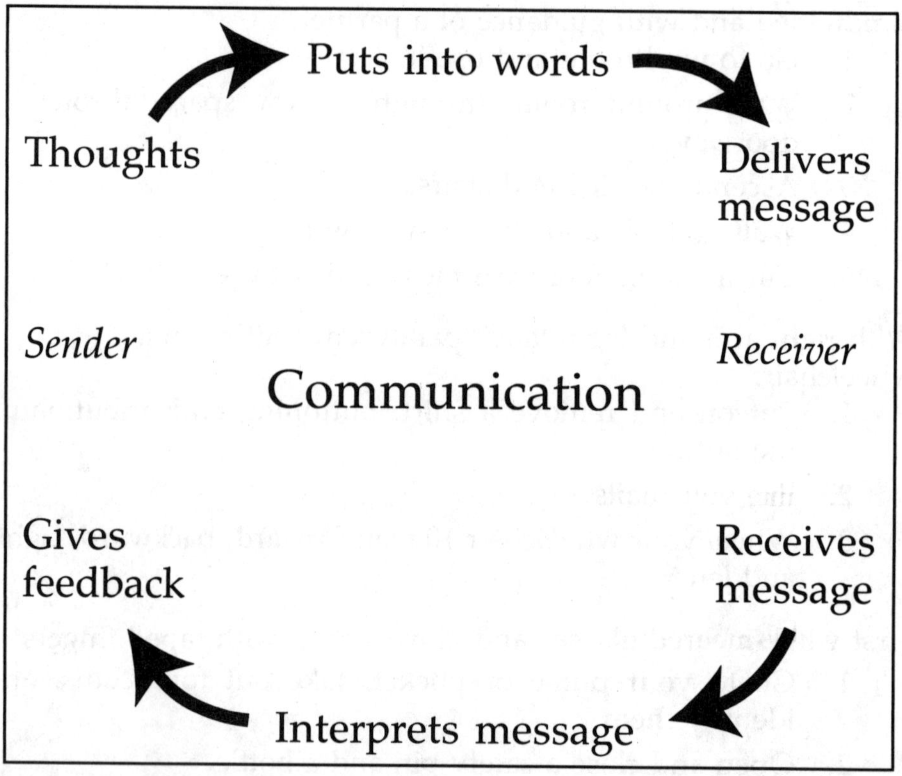

Module 2

Techniques to Improve Communication with People Who Have Hearing Loss

- Be sure you have the person's attention before beginning to speak.
- Face the person to whom you are speaking and stand reasonably close.
- Lower the pitch of your voice.
- Speak clearly and slowly.
- Use short sentences.
- Avoid background noise.
- Encourage the use of nonverbal communication, such as touch.
- Use written communication if you are unable to communicate orally.
- Do not shout; shouting makes words less clear and may cause pain.
- Do not speak with something in your mouth or with your hands over your lips.
- Give clues about what is being discussed.
- State your name before making a statement or asking a question.
- Restate your sentence when you are not understood.
- Talk toward "better" ear, for many people hear better out of one ear.
- Recognize that illness or fatigue reduces the ability of a person with a hearing impairment.
- Do not exhaust the person with irrelevant noise or chatter.
- Visual cues may assist the client; use hand gestures when appropriate; provide the opportunity for lipreading.

Module 2

Barriers to Effective Communication

Changing the Subject

It is often tempting to change a subject because the subject is uncomfortable. The client may be depressed and speaking about things that are discouraging to hear. Hang in there! He or she may need to talk about something that is deeply troubling. Changing the subject will not take the problem away. However, listening may very well ease the load.

Using Platitudes

- "Oh, you'll get over it."
- "Just make the most of it."
- "Tomorrow's another day."
- "It's God's will."

We offer these words of encouragement from time to time, and, at some point in the conversation, these reassurances may be much appreciated. However, when a person comes to you with a problem, platitudes may completely invalidate his or her feelings. Platitudes may be useful at a later point in the conversation, after the individual has had the opportunity to air his or her feelings.

Asking Closed-Ended Questions (Yes/No)

Yes/no questions are useful when you want quick answers, not when you are actually interested in a conversation. Open-ended questions are far more likely to lead to interesting dialogue. For example:

Yes/No Questions	Open-Ended Questions
• "Do you need help?"	• "How may I help you today?"
• "Would you like to go outside?"	• "Where would you like to go?"

Giving Advice

It is not our place to give advice or make recommendations. Just listening to our clients will usually help them to arrive at their own decisions.

Talking About Yourself

This is not to say that all discussion is off limits. The point is that we are there to listen to our clients, not to air our own problems.

Showing Disapproval and Passing Judgment on the Client

It is extremely important that we remain nonjudgmental of our clients. We have not walked in their shoes and cannot understand what their lives have been like.

Asking "Why" Questions

"Why" questions are a way of judging another person:

- "Why did you do that?"
- "Why are you thinking that?"

Module 2

Effective Listening Skills

- Pay attention to the speaker.
- Adopt an accepting attitude.
- Allow the speaker plenty of time.
- Stay on the subject.
- Be aware of your own emotional responses.
- Use active listening.

From Steil, L. et al. (1983). *Effective listening: Key to your success.* New York: McGraw-Hill; reprinted by permission.

Module 2

Active Listening Behaviors

Paraphrase What Has Been Said

Restating, in your own words, what the other person has said gives you a chance to check whether your understanding of what has been said is correct. It also gives the speaker a chance to correct you if you have misunderstood. You might say such things as "Do you mean that . . . ?" "I understand that you're saying. . . ."

Reflect the Speaker's Feelings

The feelings behind what is being said are often as important as the words, if not more so. Therefore, it is important to try to understand the underlying feelings, attitudes, beliefs, or values. You might make such statements as "That must have made you upset." "I imagine you were thrilled about that." "Does that worry you?"

Ask for More Information

We often need more information in order to understand what has been said. In most cases, we simply need to ask for clarification. Responses may include "I'm interested. Tell me more about that." "What happened after that?" "How did you feel when that happened?"

Nonverbally Communicate

There are many ways through which the speaker can tell whether we are listening. Through our eyes, our posture, and our gestures, we communicate our interest in what is being said.

Signs of Depression Checklist

Feelings Caused by Depression

- Extreme sadness
- Hopelessness
- Worthlessness
- Inability to enjoy life

Negative Thoughts Caused by Depression

- Fear nothing will ever get better
- Low self-esteem
- Forgetfulness
- Overwhelming guilt
- Difficulty in paying attention

Behavioral Changes Caused by Depression

- Excessive crying
- Slowness in walking, talking, and moving
- Low energy
- Poor personal appearance
- Jittery, unsettled manner
- Anxiety
- Excessive anger
- Sleep disorders

Physical Changes Caused by Depression

- Too much or too little appetite
- Weight loss
- Headaches, shortness of breath, stomachaches

Suicidal Tendencies Caused by Depression

- Thoughts about killing oneself
- Suicide threats
- Suicide attempts

Module 3

Observing a Depressed Person

- Depressed people may not take care of their hair, teeth, and skin. When questioned, they will not seem to care how they look or will say, "Oh, I just don't have the energy to do it."
- Depressed people may look sad even though they do not complain about being sad. They may cry a lot for no reason or because of sad things that happened many years ago.
- Depressed people may suddenly look old. When you try to remember what the person was like 6 months or 1 year ago, you are amazed when you realize how much he or she has aged in a short time. This is an important sign because people do not really age that much in 6 months or even a year unless they have had physical problems.
- Depressed people may want to stay in bed all the time.
- Depressed people may withdraw from activities or seem to be just going through the motions. The person does not seem to enjoy anything anymore.
- Depressed people may talk about wanting to commit suicide or say, "It would be just as well if I were hit by a car."

Module 3

Talking with a Depressed Person

Some of the issues the care provider can address with clients who resist the suggestion that they are depressed include the following:

- Specific physical changes you noticed
- Weight loss or gain
- Loss of energy
- Sleeping too much or not enough
- Crying a lot
- Not paying bills
- Not going to church (if client is a churchgoer)
- Not wanting family and friends to visit
- Not wanting to talk on the phone
- Not going out for walks
- Fears and false beliefs
- Fear people will think they are crazy
- Fear they will be locked up
- Old versus modern ideas about depression

Module 3

Ways to Help a Depressed Person

- Listen with empathy.
- Offer hope. Get the person to talk, and listen carefully to what the person says. Reassure the person over and over again that the reason he or she feels so bad is due to a medical depression that will end. Even though the depressed person will tell you that he or she does not believe things can get better, the need for hope is extremely important.
- Encourage physical activity, but do not push! For example, if a female client used to enjoy taking walks, do not expect her to initiate a walk. You will need to go and get her coat, hold it up as though you were helping her to put her coat on, and tell her, "Let's go outside for a walk." If she resists and says she cannot, you might suggest she try a short walk. Tell her that if she cannot tolerate the walk, you will be there to bring her back.
- Structure activities. Make things the person used to enjoy simpler to do. Encourage the person to do what he or she feels able to do. Be careful: Do not overwhelm the person by demanding more than he or she is able to do.
- Lighten the guilt. Recognize that depression is not something the person can change simply by being told to "shape up." Point out the person's strengths and the positive things she has done in her life before becoming depressed. When possible, identify specific positive things happening in the client's life in spite of the depression—for example, taking care of children, going to the doctor for help, making phone calls when upset, getting dressed, putting on makeup, asking for help with things difficult to do because of the depression.
- Emphasize doing with, rather than doing for. Doing everything for someone who is depressed can increase the person's feelings of helplessness and inadequacy.
- Restore areas of control. In many ways, rigidity and noncooperation are often an expression of the ways the depressed person is attempting to regain control over her life.
- Set limits. This is an act of caring that protects both you and the other person.

- Reminisce about positive past experiences. Ask direct questions about the past. Use old photos, scrapbooks, and other things from the past to help the person remember. Reminiscing may help the person to recall the past more positively and feel less worthless. Caution: When seriously depressed, some people cannot use reminiscing to feel better. If your client recalls only the pain do not pursue this option.
- Respect the person's rights to privacy and autonomy. This includes the right to make the wrong decision.
- Be watchful for signs of suicide.

Module 3

The Warning Signs of Suicide

- The older person is depressed and feels his or her situation is hopeless.
- The older person talks about wanting to end his or her life to "relieve the pain" or "solve my problems."
- The older person describes the method of suicide.
- Unusual behavior appears that is a sudden or dramatic change.
- The older person has a specific plan for suicide—the more specific the plan, the higher the risk.
- The odds are high that the suicide method the older person uses will result in his or her death.
- It is easy for the older person to obtain the means for suicide—gun, pills, car—the easier this is, the higher the risk.
- The older person becomes isolated—when a depressed, suicidal person avoids others, the risk is greater.

Module 3

Model Suicide-Prevention Policy

- Always take a suicide threat seriously.
- When reporting, be sure to state the frequency of the threats, any recent changes in the client's behavior, whether the person has a plan, and whether the person has the means to fulfill the plan.
- Steps to take when reporting:
  - √ Call supervisor.
  - √ If supervisor is not available, ask for case manager.
  - √ Report threat to a family member.
- Call 911 if the client has attempted suicide or if such an attempt seems imminent.

Module 3

Are You Under Stress?

I know I am under stress when I

- ☐ Cry more than usual
- ☐ Can't sleep
- ☐ Eat more than usual
- ☐ Am irritable
- ☐ Use alcohol or drugs
- ☐ Have "physical complaints"
- ☐ Other ________________
- ☐ Have difficulty concentrating/focusing
- ☐ Sleep more then usual
- ☐ Don't feel like eating
- ☐ Am on the move all the time
- ☐ Become overly sensitive
- ☐ Don't feel like doing anything

Stress Reducers

When I see these "symptoms," I will

- ☐ Go for a walk ______________ for ______________ minutes.
- ☐ Read a good book ____________ for ____________ minutes.
- ☐ Go shopping at _____________ for _____________ minutes.
- ☐ Exercise _________________ for _________________ minutes.
- ☐ Listen to music on the _______________________________
- ☐ Watch my favorite television program(s) ______________
- ☐ Use relaxation techniques ___________________________
- ☐ Take some time for myself by _______________________
- ☐ Do something I'm skilled at ________ for ________ minutes.
- ☐ Talk to my friend, therapist, doctor, or _________________
- ☐ Say "No" to _____________________________________
- ☐ Confront the situation by ___________________________
- ☐ Limit certain behaviors _____________________________
- ☐ Prioritize my responsibilities 1. ________________________
  2. ________________________
  3. ________________________
- ☐ Other ____

Reprinted with permission of Wellness Reproductions Inc., © 1989 (800) 669-9208.

Module 3

No One Is an "Is-Land"

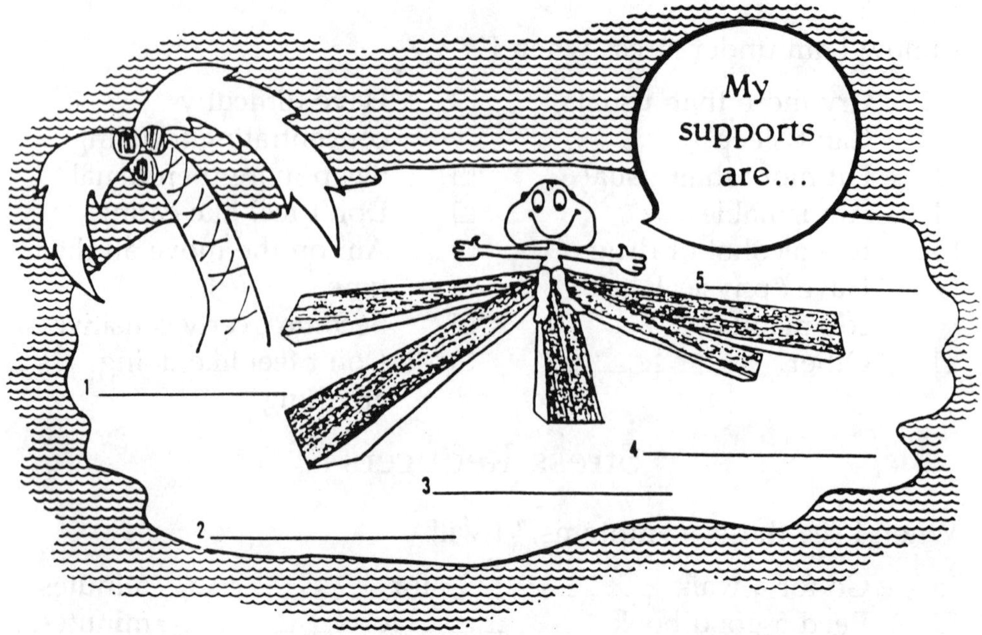

One valuable "survival skill" is having supports in our lives to help us cope. Fill in the names of your "supports" above. If you were not able to fill in all five, how or where can you find them?

___

___

___

Module 3

"I Know" About Depression Game Board

Kinds	Symptoms	Treatment	Risk Factors	Ways to Help
$100	$100	$100	$100	$100
$200	$200	$200	$200	$200
$300	$300	$300	$300	$300
$400	$400	$400	$400	$400

Module 3

"I Know" Questions

CATEGORY: KINDS

$100 Q. Is the normal depression that is part of living best described as "ups and downs," "grief," or "depression the medical illness"?

$200 Q. Can abusing alcohol cause depression?

$300 Q. Can physical illnesses cause depression?

$400 Q. Name the two symptoms that are the warning signs of depression as a medical illness.

CATEGORY: SYMPTOMS

$100 Q. Name a feeling that is a symptom of depression.

$200 Q. Name a physical complaint that is a symptom of depression.

$300 Q. Name a way a person behaves when depressed.

$400 Q. Describe a way depression affects a person's thinking.

CATEGORY: TREATMENT

$100 Q. Describe a reason why an older person may not be treated for depression.

$200 Q. Why may an older person be depressed?

$300 Q. Will depression as a medical illness go away with time?

$400 Q. Can shock treatment help a depressed person feel better?

CATEGORY: RISK FACTORS

$100 Q. Can a person die from an untreated depression?

$200 Q. Is a widow suicidal who says, "I can't wait to die so I can be with my husband!"?

$300 Q. Is an older woman suicidal when she says, "I'm tired of this pain. I'd rather be dead, and I'm going to walk in front a car some day."?

$400 Q. Can a depressed person who has memory loss be suicidal?

CATEGORY: WAYS TO HELP

$100 Q. What best conveys your concern when your client resists going to the doctor because of serious depression?

1. I am worried that you are not sleeping well. I think you need to see your doctor.
2. You shouldn't stay up all night. No wonder you feel bad; you're not getting enough sleep.

$200 Q. Which statement is the best way to encourage your client to see her doctor?

1. You mean you haven't seen your doctor yet?
2. I am concerned about you. I'll help you call your doctor.

$300 Q. Which statement best tells the person that you understand?

1. You shouldn't feel that way. It's nothing to worry about. Lots of old people have a hard time. Stop feeling sorry for yourself.
2. You sound as if you're having a difficult time. You feel very afraid and ashamed.

$400 Q. Which statement is the best way to encourage a depressed person to be physically active?

1. Get out of that chair; you need to go for a walk.
2. We are going for a walk; here is your coat.

Module 4

Memory Loss Symptoms

- Poor recall
- Reduced concentration
- Ability to calculate decreases
- "Tip of the tongue" phenomenon
- Difficulty learning new concepts
- Confusion about dates
- Loss of old skills
- Increased forgetfulness
- Poor hygiene

Module 4

Causes of Dementia

Depression

- Early symptoms look very much like dementia: poor concentration, forgetfulness, poor hygiene.
- Often misdiagnosed as dementia.
- Often viewed as a weakness rather than as a disease.
- Very treatable.

Infection

- Can cause symptoms similar to dementia.

Medication or Drug-Related Problems

- Can cause symptoms similar to dementia.
- Older people metabolize medication differently than do younger people.
- Medication combinations can cause serious memory loss problems.

Physical Disease

- Insufficient blood supply to the brain, pain, and problems associated with illnesses can cause dementia-like symptoms.

Stress and Grief

- Stress or personal loss can affect the ability to function.

Dehydration and Nutritional Deficits

- Dehydration and nutritional deficits can cause dementia—for example, a reliance on coffee and canned soups and foods, both of which are diuretics, can cause the symptoms of dementia.

Sensory Problems

- Sensory problems may mimic symptoms of dementia.
- Vision and hearing typically decline with age.

Alzheimer's Disease

- Alzheimer's disease is the most common form of dementia.
- Alzheimer's disease causes brain damage and is terminal.

- Alzheimer's disease is not a form of mental retardation or mental illness.
- Alzheimer's disease affects personality, behavior, communication, and the ability to do things, as well as memory.

Multi-Infarct Dementia (MID)

- The second most common form of dementia.
- Caused by multiple small strokes.
- Frequently occurs with Alzheimer's disease.

AIDS

- Dementia sometimes occurs in the late stages of AIDS.

Chronic Alcohol Abuse

- Korsakoff's syndrome, caused by alcohol abuse, is a type of dementia.
- Symptoms may go away if the individual stops drinking, but there is a point at which chronic alcohol abuse causes permanent damage.

Parkinson's Disease

- Parkinson's disease may cause memory loss.

Module 4

The Diagnosis of Alzheimer's Disease

- Physical exam
- Laboratory tests
- Medical histories
- Neurological exams
- Psychological and psychiatric tests
- Radiologic tests (CAT, MRI*)

*CAT, computerized axial tomography; MRI, magnetic resonance imaging

Module 4

Diagram of the Brain

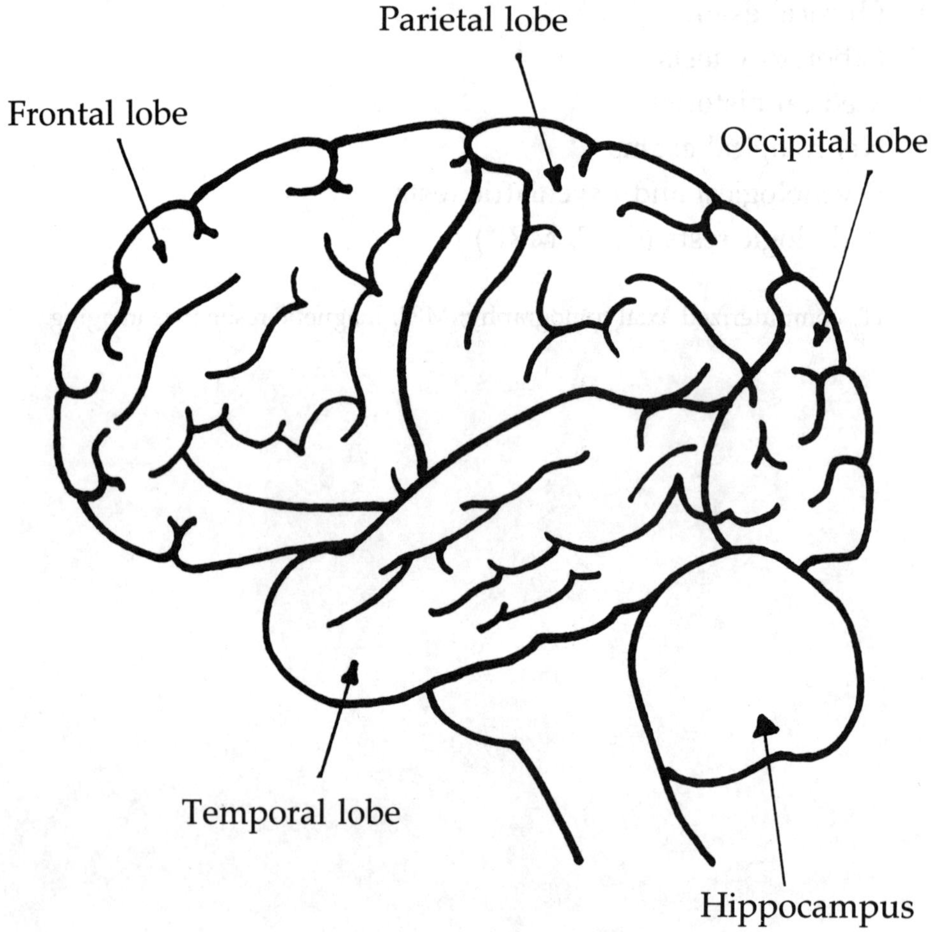

Module 4

Nerve Cells

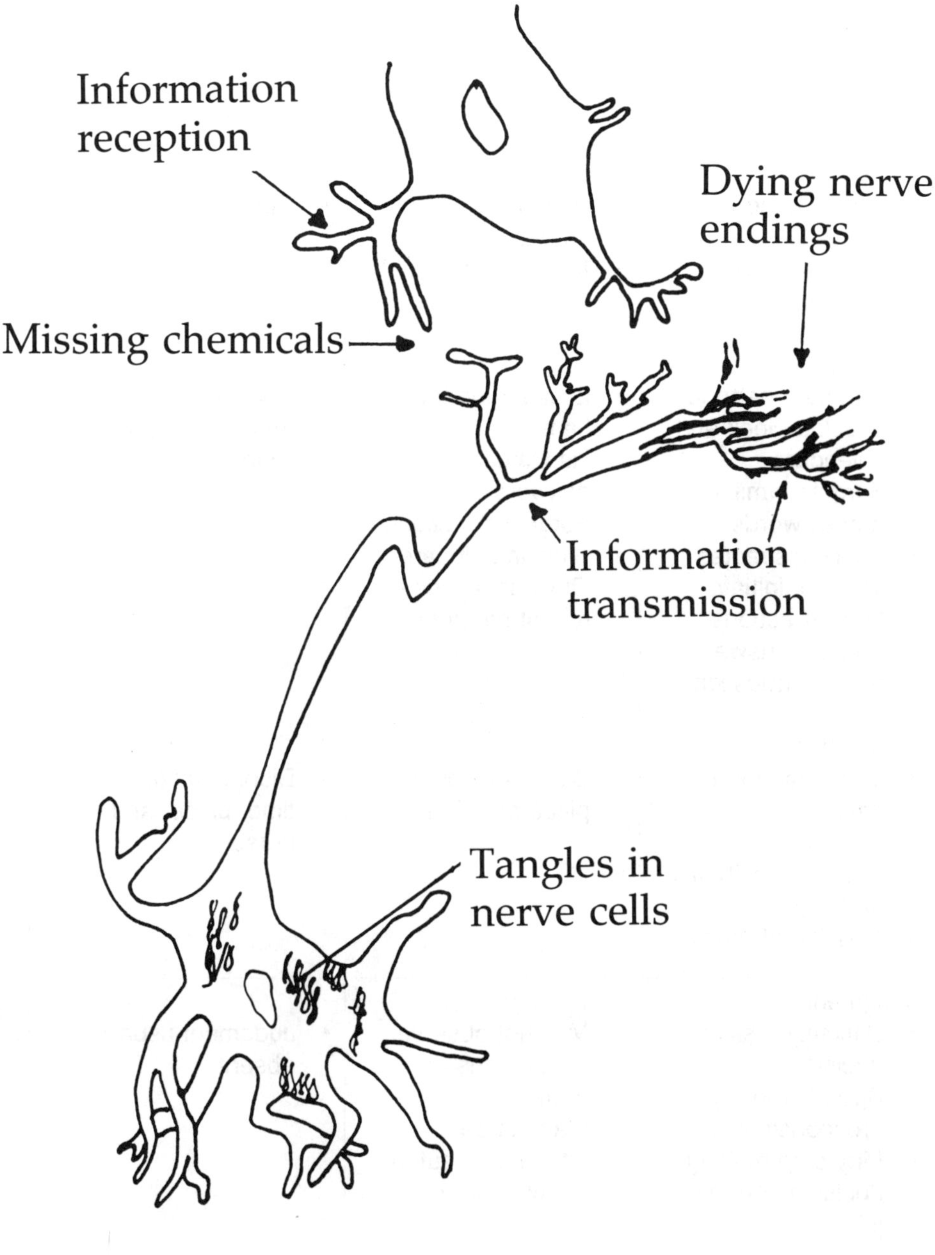

Module 4

Stages and Characteristics of Alzheimer's Disease

Stage 1	Stage 2	Stage 3
General • Appearance of stress • Exhausted yet anxious	• Symptoms more severe • Increase in loss of intellect	• Close to terminal
Memory • Frequent need to check a clock and calendar • Forgets familar names/words • Easily distracted • May not initiate familiar actions • Forgets answers/ repeats questions	• Loses important items • Hesitates with answers • Forgets directions • Slips in self-care • Obvious lapses in recent memory	• Recent and old memories very distorted
Orientation • Disorientation to time • May get lost • Confused with day and night • May forget meals	• Disorientation to place and time	• Disorientation to time, place, and person
Judgment • Difficulty making decisions • Spends money irresponsibly • May stop making decisions on the job	• May not observe precautions in traffic • May not be attentive to safety in own home	• Judgment usually absent

Learning • Difficulty concentrating • May struggle with familiar and easy tasks • Cannot make appropriate associations	• Cannot follow more than one- or two-step directions • Difficulty focusing on topic or subject	• Learning usually absent
Calculation • Problems in handling money • Frequent mistakes in bills and accounts • May lose ability to write	• Often cannot count change • Difficulty with arithmetic	• Calculation skills usually absent
Behavior • Person just not himself or herself • Loss of energy and enthusiasm • May lose interest in family affairs • May become accusative • May anger quickly • May not be as spontaneous or be slower to react	• Often does not express thoughts • May have extreme mood swings • May appear apathetic • May interpret words and places incorrectly	• May be very unaware or indifferent • May seem catatonic or coma-like • May be unable to communicate • May make only rare connections
Physical Symptoms • May have frequent physical complaints with no evidence that something is wrong • May lose weight even though appetite is still good	• May have gait and movement problems • Restless • May have an overabundance of energy • May have some physical disabilities	• Very susceptible to infection • Incontinent (both bowel and bladder) • May still be ambulatory

Module 5

Communication Problems of People with Dementia

- They are unable to express their thoughts in complete sentences.
- They lose track of their point while they are speaking.
- They get off the subject easily.
- They forget key words and names for objects.
- They cannot express their needs clearly.
- They cannot express their feelings clearly.
- They experience frustration when they are unable to speak clearly.
- They cannot understand what is being said.
- They forget English (if learned as a second language).
- They cannot follow commands (sequence of instructions).
- They experience a "tip of the tongue" feeling.
- They repeat words and phrases.
- They make up words to fill in missing phrases.
- They speak nonsense ("word salad").

Module 5

Techniques for Communicating Successfully with People with Dementia

- Speak in a normal tone of voice.
- Use the person's name frequently.
- Don't ask too many questions.
- Make questions into statements; for example, use "Let's go to the bathroom," instead of "Do you have to go to the bathroom?"
- Repeat statements or questions as often as necessary. Do not assume that understanding occurred the first time.
- Make negative statements into positive ones; for example, use "Come over here" instead of "Don't go out."
- Break directions and commands down into manageable steps.
- Wait until one step is completed before going to the next.
- Make and keep eye contact.
- Talk in a soothing, calm manner.

Module 5

Causes and Triggers of Behavior Problems in People with Dementia

- Hunger
- Medication—too little or too much
- Tiredness, fatigue, lack of energy
- Environmental stresses—too hot or too cold
- Sensory overload
- Too much going on, too many activities happening near the person, too much noise, or just too many people attempting to interact at the same time
- Time of day
- Pain or discomfort that the client is unable to name or relieve
- The need to urinate
- Unfamiliar people or surroundings
- Frustration
- Depression
- Failure

Module 5

Purposes of Leisure Activities

- To provide pleasurable passage of time
- To allow a person to pursue things that have always been of interest
- To distract a restless person
- To provide opportunities for exercise
- To increase opportunities for socialization
- To prevent behavior problems from developing
- To help a client feel like a worthwhile contributor to the world
- To encourage the highest level of independence that can be achieved
- To keep a client in touch with his or her past and present life and interests

Module 5

101 Ways to Use Capabilities

Lower Level of Ability

1. Read a story
2. Start a game of cards
3. Review family photographs
4. Read poetry
5. Hold hands and share a special moment
6. Read a newspaper aloud
7. Exercise
8. Take a walk
9. Arrange a drawer
10. Clean a closet
11. Bring your clean socks and let the client or patient help sort and fold them
12. Put on makeup and give a manicure
13. Make an indoor garden
14. Take a car ride
15. Listen to some favorite records
16. Share a family recorded message
17. Make a scrapbook
18. Share a sack lunch or box dinner from home
19. Play horseshoes—indoors or outdoors
20. Make another client or patient smile
21. Join an activity program together
22. Study the Bible
23. Clip coupons
24. Paint a picture
25. Catalog shop
26. Reminisce
27. Have a spelling bee
28. Bring something from home to share
29. Sort buttons
30. Watch a balloon sail away
31. Take family pictures
32. Read your horoscopes
33. Re-pot a plant
34. Make a grocery list and discuss prices
35. Make a Christmas list
36. Decorate a small tree
37. Give a back rub
38. Set her hair, or let the client set yours
39. Make a no-bake recipe
40. Taste something new on the market (e.g., soda or candy)
41. Play trivia
42. Practice buttoning a shirt, tying a shoe
43. Roll up skeins of yarn for future project
44. Color a picture
45. Look through a magazine
46. Start a collection to work on together
47. Have a party
48. Make a birdhouse or small project to paint
49. Review the date, time, place
50. Make a mobile for client's room
51. Bird or animal watch
52. Tear newspaper for garden mulch
53. Make a collage
54. Make ice cream
55. Pray together
56. Polish nails
57. Work on service project
58. Make some homemade lemonade
59. Pass out hugs
60. Have a tea party
61. Press flowers
62. Make holiday decorations
63. Have a picnic with all the trimmings
64. Think of 101 more things to do
65. Set a date—make plans for your next visit

HIGHER LEVEL OF ABILITY

66. Play cards
67. Work on a jigsaw puzzle
68. Work on a family tree
69. Play checkers
70. Write poetry
71. Plan the holiday meal
72. Do crossword puzzles
73. Talk about television show you have in common
74. Go for a walk
75. Make craft project
76. Make family recipe book
77. Make phone call to someone you haven't spoken with in a while
78. Polish shoes
79. Wrap a gift
80. Crochet together
81. Make party favors
82. Ask for some good old-fashioned advice
83. Sing
84. Watch and play television game show
85. What about those Bulls, Raiders, Bears, Sox, Angels?
86. Play cribbage or poker
87. Play lotto
88. Go over activity calendar and help make selections for the week
89. Make list of things you like to do
90. Write letter or card
91. Play tic-tac-toe
92. Quilt a lap blanket
93. Play bingo
94. Write an article for a newsletter
95. Travel and learn about a country through a book
96. Stencil some stationery
97. Give a book report
98. Share talent with group
99. Write your autobiography
100. Think of 101 more things to do
101. Set a date—make plans for an outing

Reprinted with permission from Rehabilitation Associates, Riverwoods, Illinois.

Module 6

Medication Use Quiz

True	False		
☐	☐	1.	Medication abuse means that the older adult does not care how he or she takes his or her medications.
☐	☐	2.	Not all medication abuse is addiction.
☐	☐	3.	Doctors always know everything about the medicines that they prescribe.
☐	☐	4.	If more than one doctor is involved with a patient, there is usually a good system of communication.
☐	☐	5.	More than a dozen people may be involved in a patient's drug therapy.
☐	☐	6.	Consumers need to learn how to inquire about what they should expect from drug therapy.
☐	☐	7.	The quality of drug therapy for older people is as clearly defined as for younger people.
☐	☐	8.	Health professionals, although often much younger than their older adult patients, understand how patients define quality of life.
☐	☐	9.	Large numbers of nursing home patients receive psychoactive drugs, even though they often do not have psychiatric diagnoses.
☐	☐	10.	Psychoactive drugs have been effective against most of the behavioral symptoms of the nursing home residents for whom the drugs are commonly prescribed.
☐	☐	11.	General Motors makes higher profits than do pharmaceutical companies.
☐	☐	12.	Some forms of noncompliance can be viewed as the patient's disagreement with the suggested drug therapy.

☐ ☐ 13. The consequences of medication abuse are likely to be more serious in an older person.

☐ ☐ 14. Up to one third of elderly admissions to hospitals are associated with drug-related problems.

☐ ☐ 15. Drug companies spend more than $2.5 billion annually to advertise their products.

Module 6

Reasons for Medication Abuse and Misuse

Polypharmacy or "doctor hopping"	Receiving prescriptions from several doctors *without* any of these doctors having knowledge of one another's prescriptions
Complicated medication regimens	Taking more than seven or eight medications
General poor communication with the doctor	Not fully understanding what the medicine is for, how it is to be taken, possible side effects, when it should be taken, and what to do if a dosage is missed
Memory impairment	Affects compliance, causing missing a dose or taking a double dose of medication
Sensory deficits	Vision or hearing problems leading to improper medication use—for example, difficulty reading small print on medication bottles, causing incorrect dosage
Self-medication	Because the pain or anxiety is not relieved with the prescribed dose, the client may take more
Mixing medications	Taking over-the-counter medications in addition to prescription medications, and neglecting to tell the doctor
Noncompliance with medication	Discontinuing medication because of unpleasant side effects or temporary relief; noncompliance can also be connected with feelings of shame or dependency about the medicine
Sharing medication or lay information	Taking someone else's medication *or* not taking own medication on someone else's advice

Medication Chart

Medication chart for:			Date:
Name of medication and dosage	Number of times per day	Time of day	Purpose
1.			
2.			
3.			
4.			
5.			
6.			
7.			
8.			

Module 6

Signs and Symptoms of Potential Medication Abuse and Misuse

- Sleep changes
- Unusual dizziness
- Mood swings
- Increased anxiety and irritability
- Confusion, especially when there was little or none before
- Ataxia (trouble in walking)
- Hostility, especially if this represents a radical change
- Loss of balance
- Defensive attitude
- Missed doctor's appointments
- Appetite changes
- Groggy or lethargic
- Difficulty managing pain

Module 6

Medication Abuse and Misuse—How To Help

- The care provider is responsible for keeping an eye out for clues (actions, symptoms, or communication) and for reporting to a supervisor.
- Build rapport and trust with a client. This helps develop a relationship in which the provider can pick up verbal clues.
- Always let clients know that confidentiality will be respected but that, in the best interest of their health and safety, information will be shared with their health care team. This is particularly true if a client says, "I'll tell you this if you promise not to tell anyone."
- Your supervisor can involve other members of the health care team. A nurse and/or doctor can work with the client to educate the person on proper usage of medication. Sometimes misuse happens as a result of misunderstanding.
- If an older person is having problems keeping track of a complicated medication regimen, ask the nurse to contact the physician for an easier one.
- Be aware of other ways abuse and misuse can happen: taking someone else's medications, taking too much or too little medicine, stopping medicine on one's own, combining medications and alcohol.
- Look carefully at possible medication interaction. Notify a supervisor, a nurse, or the doctor involved, or encourage the client and family to do so.
- If possible, help clients correct sensory deficits—for example, make sure that they wear their glasses and hearing aids.

Module 6

Common Medication Abbreviations

a.c.	before meals	PO	by mouth
ad lib	freely, as desired	PR	by rectum
b.i.d.	two times a day	PRN	when required
c̄	with	q	every
caps.	capsule	q.d.	every day
gtt	a drop	q.h.	every hour
hr	hour	q.h.s.	every night
h.s.	hour of sleep, bedtime	q.i.d.	four times a day
i	one	q.o.d.	every other day
ii	two	s̄	without
O.D.	right eye	s̄s̄	one half
O.S.	left eye	tab.	tablet
os	mouth	t.i.d.	three times a day
p.c.	after meals	ung.	ointment

Module 7

Beliefs About Alcohol Problems

	True	False	
1.	☐	☐	Alcoholism is a sign of moral weakness.
2.	☐	☐	The alcoholic is a street bum, down and out.
3.	☐	☐	Older women do not have alcohol problems.
4.	☐	☐	A person has to drink a lot and often to develop a drinking problem.
5.	☐	☐	Alcohol helps lift a person's mood.
6.	☐	☐	Alcohol helps digestion.
7.	☐	☐	Alcohol helps a person sleep.
8.	☐	☐	Drinking is an older person's last remaining pleasure. It is wrong to take it away.
9.	☐	☐	A person has to "hit bottom" before he or she can be helped.
10.	☐	☐	Older people who have an alcohol problem *cannot* be successfully treated.
11.	☐	☐	Treatment is just to stop drinking.

Source: Schmall, V. L., & Stiehl, R. E. (1990). *Winter comforts.* Corvallis, OR: Oregon State University Extension Service. Reprinted with permission.

Module 7

Facts About Alcoholism

- Rates of alcoholism vary in the older adult.
- Generally, alcohol use tends to decrease with age.
- Although the rate of substance abuse is lower in older adults, alcohol is the most abused substance.
- Widowers have the highest rate of alcoholism; never-married women have the lowest rate.
- Alcohol use onset after age 65 is often connected with severe chronic illness, coping with a significant loss, and/or traumatic life experiences.
- From 500,000–2 million older Americans have some type of drinking problem.
- Of fatal motor vehicle accidents, 12% are related to alcohol abuse and involve persons 65 and older.

Module 7

Barriers to Treatment

- Signs and symptoms of alcohol abuse in the older adult may go unrecognized because these symptoms mimic other aging-related problems.
- The social stigma of alcoholism will often cause people to avoid talking about it.
- Feelings of helplessness occur on the part of us, the professionals: How should we handle this?
- It can be difficult to deal with the attitudes of the families of these clients.
- The feeling often arises on the part of both families and professionals that older people should be able to do as they like with the remainder of their life.
- Older people who abuse alcohol are more isolated.
- Lack of financial resources or lack of knowledge about available treatment choices keeps people from seeking help.
- Health professionals may have misconceptions about treatment of alcoholism in older individuals.
- Our own attitudes and beliefs, including a possible fear of addressing this issue, may keep us from helping the client.

Module 7

Alcohol Abuse in Later Life

- Early-onset alcoholics or chronic alcoholics are actually survivors of alcohol problems that began in their youth.
- Late-onset alcoholics start drinking after the age of 40.
- Losses people experience as they age contribute to depression and can lead to increased alcohol use. These include death of a spouse, death or relocation of lifelong friends, retirement and/or loss of job status, financial insecurity, diminishing ability to drive, and deteriorating physical health.
- Late-onset alcoholism may be related to loneliness, boredom, and lack of purpose.
- Although loneliness and isolation can contribute to the problem of alcoholism, recent evidence suggests that problems with alcohol often develop in retirement communities where social drinking may be prevalent.
- Physical illness and depression related to a decline in physical health can lead to alcoholism.

Module 7

Special Risk Factors

- Age-related physical changes put the older alcoholic at special risk.
- Metabolic breakdown of alcohol in the body is less efficient in older adults, resulting in higher blood alcohol levels than would be seen in a younger individual consuming the same amount of alcohol.
- The brain and central nervous system of an older individual are much more sensitive to alcohol, resulting in a diminished tolerance. Alcohol depresses the central nervous system. It can cause depression or make an existing depression worse. Alcohol also accelerates the loss of brain cells.
- Older individuals who abuse alcohol are much more likely to develop gastrointestinal problems. Alcohol abuse increases the secretion of digestive enzymes, causing heartburn, ulcers, gastritis, and intestinal bleeding.
- Even small amounts of alcohol in an older person can decrease cardiac output and coronary circulation. Chronic drinking increases the risk of heart disease. Alcohol will make high blood pressure worse.
- Older people with preexisting conditions, such as lung disease and diabetes, can be especially at risk.
- Alcohol ingestion is especially serious for clients who take prescription medications. Medications can intensify the effects of alcohol, leading to rapid intoxication. Conversely, alcohol can decrease the effectiveness of the medication.
- Alcohol combined with sleeping pills can severely depress the central nervous system, leading to coma or death.
- An older alcoholic who stops drinking suddenly can face life-threatening consequences.

Module 7

Signs of an Alcohol Problem

- Abrupt changes in an individual's behavior
- Frequent accidents such as burns, falls, and abnormal bruising
- Weight loss and decreased appetite
- Pale, yellowish, or unhealthy-looking skin
- Frequent napping and complaints of disturbed sleep
- Constant fatigue
- Hangovers and blackouts
- Confusion
- Frequent headaches
- Deterioration in grooming and housekeeping
- Alcohol noted on breath
- Hiding liquor bottles

Module 7

Interventions and Treatment

- Build trust and rapport through day-to-day contact and conversation.
- Share concerns/suspicions with supervisor.
- Have intervention coordinated by a trained professional.
- Use a loving, gentle approach where concern is expressed and the client is encouraged to seek help.
- Encourage client to share some feelings, especially regarding illness and losses.
- Be nonjudgmental.
- Approach in the least intrusive manner.
- Promote alcoholic day-treatment centers.

Module 7

Recognizing an Alcohol Problem: Changes in Drinking Patterns

- ☐ The person is drinking a larger quantity than before
- ☐ The person is drinking more often
- ☐ The person is drinking at different times or places
- ☐ The person is drinking in the morning
- ☐ The person drinks alone more often
- ☐ The person organizes activities around drinking
- ☐ The person seems preoccupied with drinking
- ☐ The person makes excuses about drinking
- ☐ The person smells of alcohol
- ☐ The person is protective of alcohol supply
- ☐ The person sneaks drinks
- ☐ The person drinks despite health problems
- ☐ The person looks intoxicated
- ☐ The person regrets or forgets things he or she did while drinking
- ☐ The person is unwilling to talk about his or her drinking

Source: Adapted with permission from Schmall, V. L., & Stiehl, R. E. (1990). *Winter Comforts.* Corvallis, OR: Oregon State University Extension Service.

Module 7

Recognizing an Alcohol Problem: Changes in Behavior

- ☐ The person neglects personal appearance
- ☐ The person neglects home, bills, pets
- ☐ The person has cigarette burns on clothing, furniture, self
- ☐ The person uses perfume or breath fresheners excessively
- ☐ The person has erratic sleep patterns
- ☐ The person displays increased irritability, agitation, anxiety
- ☐ The person harbors unreasonable resentments
- ☐ The person loses interest in activities and people
- ☐ The person neglects eating
- ☐ The person displays personality changes
- ☐ The person has recurring episodes of memory loss
- ☐ The person has frequent, unusual, or neglected injuries
- ☐ The person has bruises, especially at furniture height
- ☐ The person displays slowed thought process
- ☐ The person withdraws from social relationships
- ☐ The person has suicidal thoughts or makes suicide attempts
- ☐ The person suffers frequent falls

Source: Adapted with permission from Schmall, V. L., & Stiehl, R. E. (1990). *Winter Comforts*. Corvallis, OR: Oregon State University Extension Service.

Module 7

Recognizing an Alcohol Problem: Changes in Physical Condition

- ☐ The person has general physical deterioration
- ☐ The person has slurred speech
- ☐ The person has weight gain or loss
- ☐ The person has tremors
- ☐ The person has skin changes (sallow or flushed)
- ☐ The person has yellow or bloodshot eyes
- ☐ The person has fatigue
- ☐ The person has leg cramps
- ☐ The person has malnutrition
- ☐ The person has blurred vision
- ☐ The person has edema (swelling, a bloated look)
- ☐ The person has blackouts
- ☐ The person has chronic gastric problems
- ☐ The person has hypertension (especially if no previous history)
- ☐ The person has heart arrhythmia
- ☐ The person has sexual impotence
- ☐ The person has urinary incontinence

Source: Adapted with permission from Schmall, V. L., & Stiehl, R. E. (1990). *Winter Comforts*. Corvallis, OR: Oregon State University Extension Service.

Types of Abuse Reported

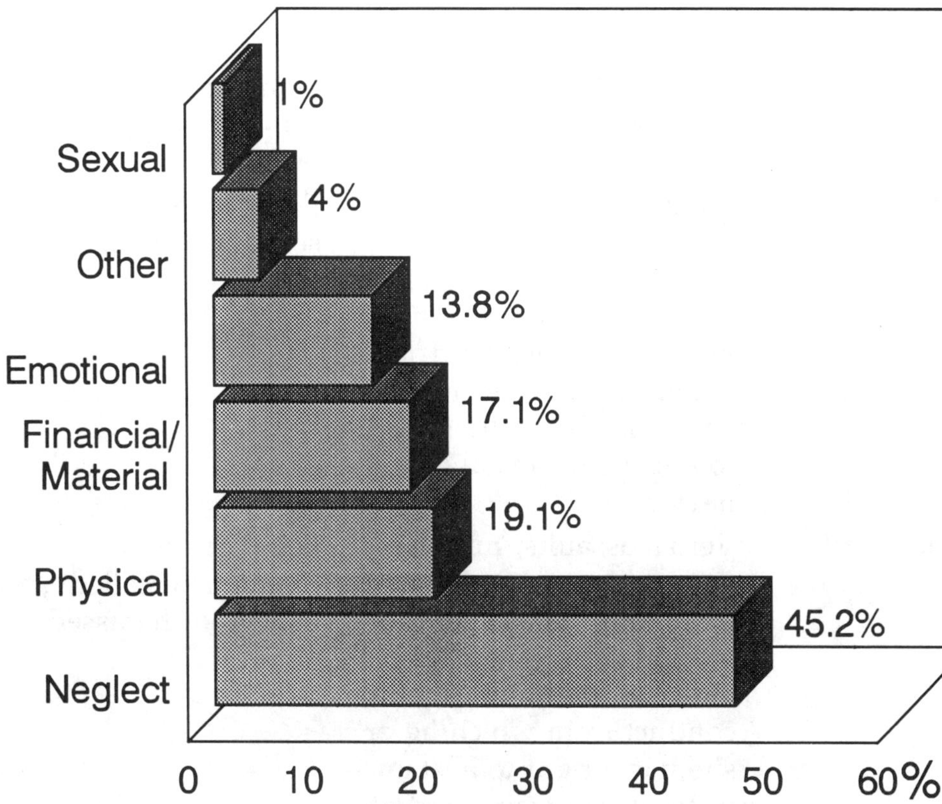

Source: Totara, 1993.

Module 8

Types of Abuse, Neglect, and Exploitation

Physical	The inflicting of physical pain or injury on an older person	Being handled roughly, slapped, or hit
Sexual	Touching, fondling, or any other sexual activity with an older person when the older person is unable to understand, unwilling to consent, threatened, or physically forced to engage in sexual behavior	Being forced to be sexually intimate
Emotional	Verbal assaults, humiliation, and threats of maltreatment, harassment, or intimidation to compel the older person to engage in conduct from which he or she has a right to abstain or to refrain from conduct in which he or she has a right to engage	Being insulted, threatened, called names, or harassed
Confinement	Restraining or isolating an older person for other than medical reasons	Tying an older person to a bed or chair to prevent him or her from wandering when he or she is not being supervised
Passive neglect	Another person willfully withholding from or refusing to provide an eligible adult with the necessities of life, including, but not limited to, food, clothing, shelter, and medical care	Refusing to hire a cleaning service, neglecting to pay bills on time, and purchasing small amounts of food or poor-quality food

Willful deprivation	Willfully keeping from or denying older people, disabled people, or those in poor health the care they need; this can include denying them medication, medical care, shelter, food, therapeutic devices, or other physical assistance	Being denied food, clothing, shelter, medical care, or social contact
Financial exploitation	The misuse or withholding of an older person's resources by another person (to the disadvantage of the older person) and/or the profit or advantage of a person other than the older person	Being forced to sign over money (Social Security checks, pension checks, savings accounts) or property (the victim's home or other real estate)

Module 8

Abuser's Relationship to Victim

(70% of abusers are family members)

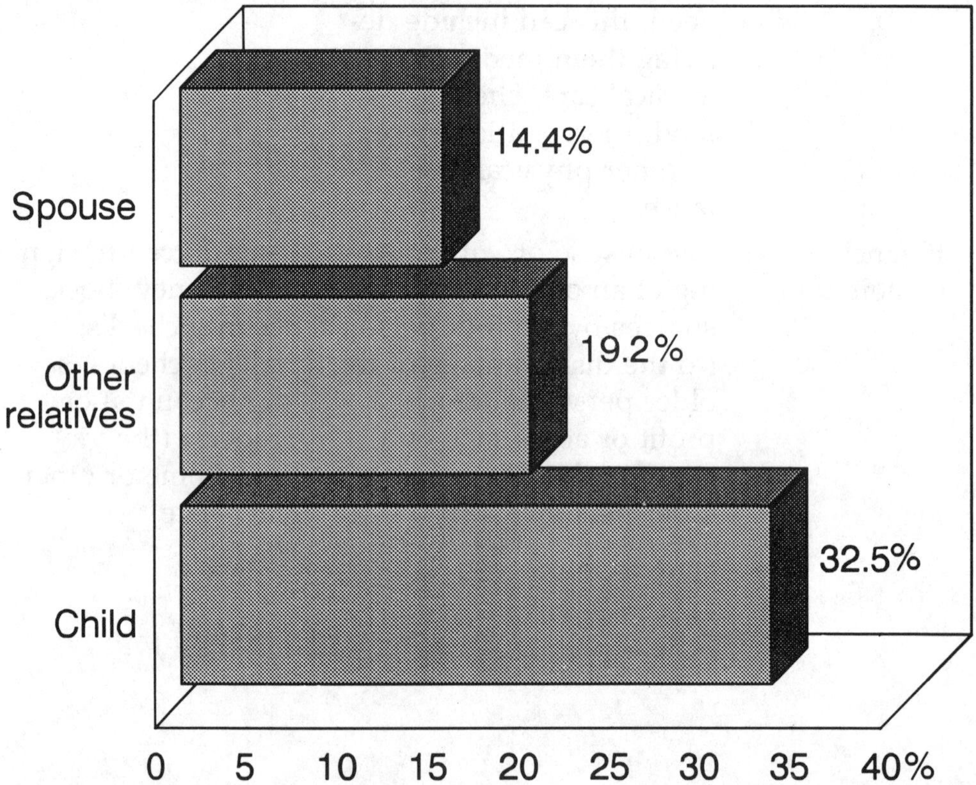

Source: Totara, 1993.

Abusers

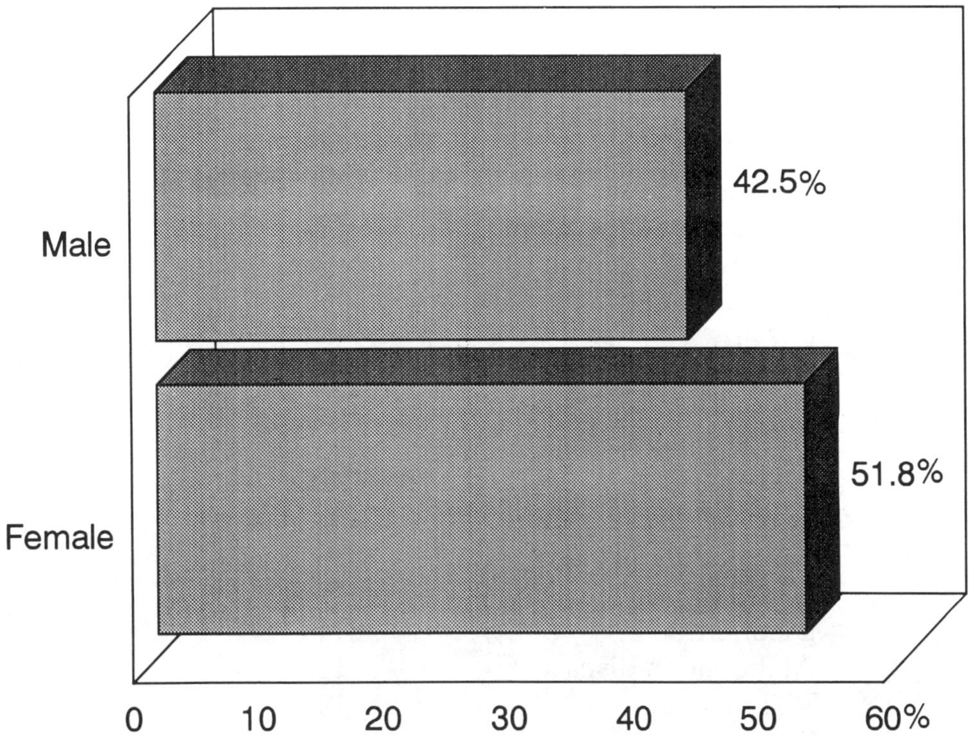

Source: Totara, 1993.

Module 8

Characteristics of the Abuser and the Victim

Abuser

Factor	**Frequency (%)**
Substance abuser	24
Financially dependent	14
Functionally impaired	3
Mental illness	3
Other	13
None identified	52

Victim

Factor	**Frequency (%)**
Functionally impaired	30
Nonambulatory	18
Hearing loss	15
Disoriented	14
Alzheimer's disease	13
Vision loss	13
Speech loss	11
Substance abuse	9
Other	14
None mentioned	24

Module 8

Victims

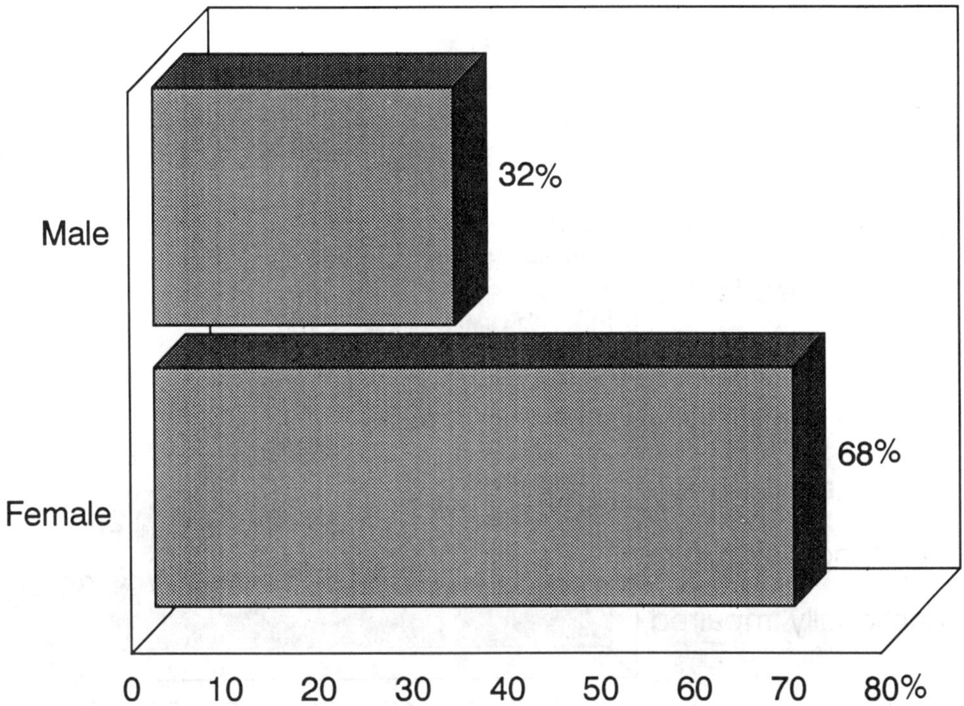

Source: Totara, 1993.

Victims

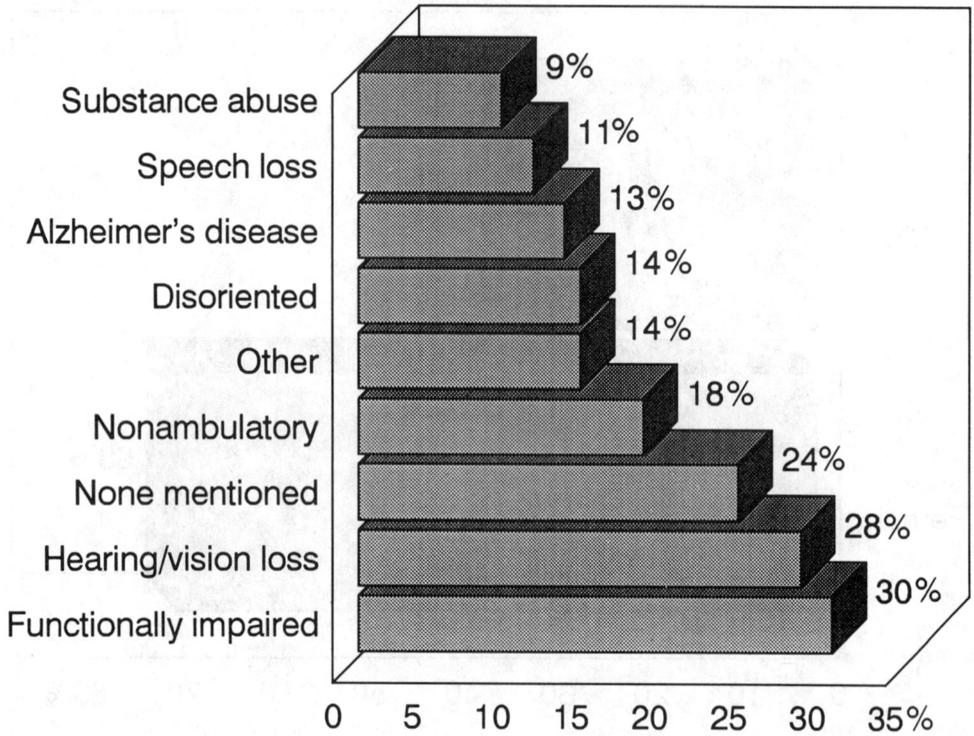

Source: Totara, 1993.

Module 8

Signs of Physical Abuse

- Bruises (sometimes shaped like an object), welts, discoloration found bilaterally on upper arms, clustered on the trunk, or all over body area
- Evidence of inadequate care (e.g., bedsores that have not been treated), soiled clothing and bed linens, lack of bandages or stitches when indicated, evidence of broken bones
- Poor skin hygiene, absence of hair, hemorrhaging (bruising) below the scalp
- Burns from cigarettes, acids, caustics; friction from ropes or other bindings
- Signs of confinement: client tied to furniture or bathroom fixtures, locked in a room
- Lack of necessary appliances (e.g., walker, cane, or bedside commode); lack of heat, food, or water; unsafe conditions

Module 8

Abusive Behaviors of Family Members or Caregiver

- The older person may not be able to speak for herself or to see others without her children present.
- There are attitudes of indifference or anger toward the older person or an obvious absence of assistance.
- Family members blame the older person for problem behaviors (e.g., incontinence, forgetfulness).
- Aggressive behavior is shown toward the older person (e.g., threats, insults, or harassment).
- There is a previous history of abuse in the family (e.g., domestic violence, child abuse).
- There is withholding of security or affection.
- Problems with alcohol, drugs, or mental illness are observed.
- The family member and/or the older person is socially isolated.
- Conflicting accounts of incidents are offered by family, supporters, and victim.
- Family members display unwillingness or reluctance to comply with the care plan.

Module 8

Indicators of Financial Exploitation

- A caregiver or family member with access to an older person's money appears to use the funds for his or her own purchases rather than for the older person, causing unpaid bills, overdue rent, and so on.
- An older adult does not have adequate food, clothing, or personal care items when there appears to be enough money to provide them.
- An older person is grossly overcharged for rent or services.
- An older person complains of deception or theft of property or funds.

Module 9

Values Clarification Exercise

1. What motivated you to accept a job in which you take care of older people? Were there particular values that you held that led you to do this kind of work? If so, what were they?

____

____

____

____

____

____

2. When caring for an older person, have you ever been in a situation that was difficult for you because a particular value that you hold was called into conflict? What was the situation? What was the value that was called into conflict? Why was it called into conflict?

____

____

____

____

____

____

Module 9

Confidentiality Vignette 1

Mary has just started working for Mrs. Himmel. Mrs. Himmel is a nice, friendly woman for whom Mary does some homemaking tasks. Sometimes Mary has a few free minutes, and the two of them sit and chat. In making conversation, Mrs. Himmel asks about some of Mary's other clients.

Mary tells her about Mrs. Tewey, a client she works for in the mornings before she comes to work for Mrs. Himmel. She tells Mrs. Himmel that the situation with Mrs. Tewey is difficult because Mr. Tewey has Alzheimer's disease. He swears, is incontinent, is very confused and forgetful, and sometimes even hits Mrs. Tewey.

When Mary saw Mrs. Tewey the next time, Mrs. Tewey was furious with her. Apparently, Mrs. Tewey and Mrs. Himmel know each other from church. When Mrs. Himmel heard about how bad Mrs. Tewey's situation was, she called her in concern. Mrs. Tewey was terribly embarrassed. While she has shared with Mrs. Himmel and other members of her church that her husband has Alzheimer's disease, she has not let them know about his behavior problems. Her husband has been a very respected member of the church, and she feels he would be embarrassed if anyone knew what he had become like because of his condition.

Mrs. Tewey is so embarrassed that she does not want to go back to her own church.

Discussion Questions

1. What do you think about what happened?
2. How could Mary have better handled Mrs. Himmel's questions about her other cases?
3. If you were Mrs. Tewey, would you have felt the way she did? Why or why not?
4. If you do not think you would have reacted the way Mrs. Tewey did, do you feel she had a right to be upset?

Module 9

Confidentiality Vignette 2

Mr. Grossman, 82 years old, expressed concerns about killing himself to his care provider on numerous occasions. Mr. Grossman was severely depressed, physically ill, and had a very unhealthy relationship with his family. Mr. Grossman stored a gun on a shelf in his bedroom closet.

The care provider tried to talk to Mr. Grossman about the value of life. Months went by, and Mr. Grossman became more definite in his statements about suicide. The caregiver finally reported this case to the supervisor during an in-service training on suicide.

A social worker was immediately assigned to this case. Mr. Grossman was very upset that the care provider, whom he had known for several years, would break his confidence. Mr. Grossman no longer wanted her to return.

Discussion Questions

1. Was the caregiver right to be concerned about Mr. Grossman?
2. Should the caregiver have reported the case to the supervisor?
3. Should the caregiver have talked to Mr. Grossman about his suicidal thoughts? Should the caregiver have spoken with Mr. Grossman's family?
4. How would you have handled this situation?

Module 9

Care Provider Code of Ethics

Confidentiality: the act of keeping something private or secret

Examples of Ethical Behavior:

1. Not discussing my client's finances with other clients.

2. ______________________________

3. ______________________________

4. ______________________________

5. ______________________________

6. ______________________________

Module 9

Care Provider Code of Ethics

Elder Abuse: mistreatment (verbal, emotional, or physical)

Examples of Ethical Behavior:

1. Discussing "suspicious" bruises or cuts with my supervisor.
2. ______________________________
3. ______________________________
4. ______________________________
5. ______________________________
6. ______________________________

Module 9

Care Provider Code of Ethics

Substance Abuse: mistreatment of body with alcohol or drugs

Examples of Ethical Behavior:

1. Let supervisor know about client's misuse of medications.

2. ____________________

3. ____________________

4. ____________________

5. ____________________

6. ____________________

Module 9

Care Provider Code of Ethics

Sexuality: the state of being physically intimate

Examples of Ethical Behavior:

1. Not accepting sexual advances from a client.

2. ______________________________

3. ______________________________

4. ______________________________

5. ______________________________

6. ______________________________

Module 9

Care Provider Code of Ethics

Death, Dying, Suicide: the ending of life

Examples of Ethical Behavior:

1. Need to report client's discussion of suicide plans to supervisor.
2. ______________________________
3. ______________________________
4. ______________________________
5. ______________________________
6. ______________________________

Module 9

Care Provider Code of Ethics

Money and Gifts: expressions of thanks

Examples of Ethical Behavior:

1. Not accepting monetary gifts from clients.
2. ______________________________
3. ______________________________
4. ______________________________
5. ______________________________
6. ______________________________

Module 9

Sexuality and Older People

Myth: Older people do not have the ability to engage in sexual relations.

Fact: While some illnesses may interfere with sexual performance, if the older person (as well as his or her partner) is reasonably healthy, sexual relations are possible into the 70s, 80s, and even 90s.

Myth: Older people are not interested in sex.

Fact: Overall, there is a decline in sexual interest with increasing age, but sexuality holds a place of great importance for most older persons.

Myth: People who engaged in sex regularly when they were younger cannot continue this pattern into old age.

Fact: Sexual patterns tend to persist throughout the lifetime, and those who were sexually active in their younger years are the most active in their later years.

Myth: Older people do not have alternative lifestyles; they are not homosexual, and they do not have sex outside of marriage.

Fact: While they tend to be more "closeted" than their younger counterparts, older homosexuals certainly exist. There are also many older persons who engage in sexual relations with partners to whom they are not married.

Module 9

Sexuality Vignette

A care provider goes to the home of Mr. and Mrs. Walker to provide a break for Mrs. Walker. Mrs. Walker goes out shopping for a couple of hours while the caregiver takes care of Mr. Walker, who is 85 years old and disabled. Mr. Walker compliments the caregiver on how beautiful she is. She just smiles, thinking that "it's a cute thing for this older gentleman to say." On the next visit, Mr. Walker says, "Would you ever go out with a guy like me?" The caregiver giggles and says, "Sure! You're cute!" During the following visit, he makes his move. He grabs at her and tries to kiss her.

The care provider is outraged. She calls her supervisor and wants to be taken off the case. What went wrong?

Module 9

Acceptance of Money and Gifts

- Avoid asking for money or gifts from clients.
- Do not accept money or gifts from confused clients. Notify the family or the supervisor if you are offered money.
- Avoid managing the client's money in any way. Do not offer financial advice.
- Do not argue with clients about money. If the client refuses to pay, notify the family or the supervisor.
- Do not spend your own money on groceries, etc., unless you have worked out a plan for this with the family and social worker.
- Keep an accurate record on time sheets.
- Keep receipts of all items purchased for clients.
- Do not borrow money from clients.

Module 9

Money and Gifts Vignettes

Ms. Douglas has received shopping services for the last 10 years from the same care provider. During that 10-year period, Ms. Douglas has suffered a stroke, which caused some memory impairment, and has had cataract surgery on both eyes.

The caregiver was so comfortable with Ms. Douglas that she often would not record her payment in the worker receipt book. On this particular day, she reported to Ms. Douglas's home at the usual time and obtained the shopping list. Ms. Douglas gave her two $10 bills.

When the care provider returned, she handed Ms. Douglas 48 cents in change and placed the groceries on the kitchen counter. The caregiver said the bill came to $19.52.

After the care provider left for the day, the client called the supervisor and reported that she had given the caregiver a $20 and a $10. She accused the care provider of keeping the $10 bill for herself.

During investigation of the complaint made by Ms. Douglas, the supervisor asked the caregiver for a copy of the receipt for proof of purchase, but she had lost the receipt. The supervisor then asked for the receipt for any financial transactions that took place in the field that day, but one had never been filled out.

The supervisor knew that Ms. Douglas was suffering from memory impairment and that the care provider was innocent, but the worker did not follow proper guidelines to protect herself against accusations of theft.

What would you do?

Mrs. Carter has received in-home services for at least 3 years from the same caregiver, who knows exactly what Mrs. Carter wants done in her home. One day, when the care provider was ready to go, it started to rain heavily.

Mrs. Carter insisted that the caregiver take the raincoat located in the hall closet and keep it for other rainy days. Two weeks later the client reported to the supervisor that her raincoat was missing and that it was last seen on the day that the care provider was in her home.

What would you do?

Module 10

Stages of Grief

Denial and Isolation

The first reaction a person has is to try to push the knowledge away. Also, it is normal for the terminally ill person and the family to struggle with feelings of isolation.

Anger: "Why Me?"

This is a very common question terminally ill people and their family members ask when they start to come to terms with the reality that the person is going to die.

Bargaining

People often try to bargain by making promises to God or some higher power to allow them to live.

Depression

It is normal for terminally ill people and their families to experience a sadness so deep that, at times, they may not be able to perform even the simplest tasks.

Acceptance

The final step in the grieving process is acceptance. People may not need to talk a lot about all the thoughts and feelings they are experiencing, but when they talk about their illness and eventual death, there is a different feeling . . . a kind of a calm.

Module 10

The Special Needs of Terminally Ill People

- To be listened to attentively
- To talk about the meaningful times in their lives
- To review the happy times of the past
- To talk about their families and their families' future
- To talk with someone who is comfortable having an open and frank discussion of death-related issues
- To put their practical affairs in order
- To be physically comfortable
- To have control over when and how physical care will be provided
- To have an explanation of what is being done during the provision of physical care
- To have comforting items, such as pictures of family members, sentimental things, favorite book, and jewelry, near them
- To have someone physically present to be there and care
- To have calm caregivers
- To have privacy
- To maintain a personal sense of dignity
- To be treated with respect
- To be able to participate in family rituals and customs
- To be able to pursue their religious beliefs or philosophy that enables the dying person to understand death

Module 11

Stress

Stressor

Stress Reaction

Stress Mediators

- Ways of looking at stressor
- Ways of looking at ourselves
- Ways of coping with stress
- Outside support to help with stressor
- Physical and psychological conditions

Module 11

Stress-Related Diseases

- Heart disease
- Hypertension
- Kidney disease
- Arteriosclerosis
- Chronic backache
- Gastritis
- Migraines
- Psoriasis
- Eczema
- Cold sores
- Shingles
- Hives
- Ulcers

Module 11

Stress-Related Body Changes

- Heart beats faster
- Blood pressure rises
- Muscles tense to prepare for action
- Digestion stops
- Saliva dries up
- Sugars and fats are released into the bloodstream
- Breathing accelerates
- Blood-clotting mechanisms are activated
- Red blood cells increase
- Pupils dilate
- Senses are heightened
- Bowel and bladder muscles are weakened
- Perspiration increases
- Adrenaline and endomorphin are released into the bloodstream
- Endomorphin blocks pain, sometimes resulting in a feeling of euphoria

Module 11

Signs of Stress

Physical

- Headaches
- Dry mouth or throat
- Neck pain
- Backaches
- Constipation
- Stomach pains
- Rashes and hives
- Heart palpitations
- Excessive sweating
- Sexual problems
- Swollen joints
- Trembling
- Twitches
- Difficulty in swallowing
- Difficulty in breathing
- Dizziness
- Muscle aches
- Indigestion
- Diarrhea
- Chest pains
- Frequent urination
- Insomnia
- High blood pressure
- Increased allergies
- Accident proneness
- Facial or jaw pain
- Tongue ulcers
- Speech problems
- Weakness
- Nausea or vomiting
- Weight gain or loss
- Heartburn
- Cold hands/feet
- Excessive sleeping
- Difficulty in sleeping
- Chronic fatigue
- Frequent colds or flu
- Menstrual irregularities

Emotional

- Depression
- Memory loss
- Overexcitability
- Impulsive behavior
- Neurotic behavior
- Indecisiveness
- Suicidal tendencies
- Lack of interest in sex
- Irritability
- Restlessness
- Nervousness
- Anger
- Withdrawal
- Feelings of panic
- Confused
- Difficulty in concentrating
- Anxiety
- Nightmares
- Frustration
- Feeling helpless
- Disorientation
- Frequent crying
- Loss of control

Behavioral

- Pacing the floor
- Gnashing or grinding teeth
- Foot or finger tapping
- Hair pulling or twisting
- Increased medication use
- Chronic procrastination
- Increased alcohol consumption
- Compulsive eating/ compulsive dieting
- Nervous laughter
- Wrinkling forehead
- Chronic tardiness
- Increased smoking
- Nail biting
- Sudden change in social habits
- Loss of interest in appearance

Module 11

Ways to Cope with Stress

Withdrawal

Withdrawal is a style of avoiding, fearing, or otherwise putting off action that would reduce pressure. Withdrawal means you are not taking risks, making changes, or meeting responsibility. This leads to worry, depression, fear, and frustration.

Ways to Change

Make a list of the important things you have to do and reasons for not doing them. Then think of ways to change the reasons. Face the task directly, and set a checklist for action. Take time to relax. Imagine doing the task step by step. Imagine doing the task well and feeling good about it. Create rewards for yourself at each step, including completion. Think about why you find it difficult to begin the task. Ask yourself what would be the worst that could happen. Ask yourself if you really should be doing the task. Resistance is a signal that the job may not be right for you.

Helplessness

Helplessness is the feeling that you cannot do things or that what you can do will not make a difference. It is usually paired with hopelessness. Helplessness is a self-defeating circle. Changing helplessness begins by looking at the negative things you say to yourself.

Ways to Change

Think about the things you say to yourself, and try new ways to find your strengths. Lower your expectations of yourself. It is all right to make mistakes and correct them. Take action; any small step is better than doing nothing.

Internalizing

Internalizers keep things to themselves. Holding in feelings, resentment, and worries can lead to headaches, stomachaches, and other ailments that can cause an emotional outburst. To change this behavior, one needs to be aware of these feelings as they are building up and find good ways to express them.

Ways to Change

Practice body awareness. Note what feelings are building up. Sometimes just being aware of your feelings is enough to help reduce the stress. Think of your reasons for not sharing your feelings. You may find that when you say them to yourself, your reasons are not so scary. Express how you feel without expecting the other person to do something about it.

Emotional Outbursts

Emotional outbursts are the long-term outcomes of internalizing. They release tension in a safe environment and often involve shifting blame and responsibility to another person. Though tension is relieved, the source of frustration is unchanged.

Ways to Change

Become aware of emotions as they emerge. Ask yourself why you feel that way and what you can do to change it. Take action before you have a blow-up.

Overcontrolling

Keeping things under control is one of the most important and successful methods of stress management. However, overcontrolling makes stress worse because it is impossible to control everything.

Ways to Change

Evaluate which tasks can be dropped and which can be given to others. Look at why losing control is scary, and take steps to change those feelings.

Module 11

Your Best Qualities

Write down five of your best qualities

1. ______________________________

   ____

2. ______________________________

   ____

3. ______________________________

   ____

4. ______________________________

   ____

5. ______________________________

   ____

Module 11

Time Management

- Take some time—no matter how little you have—to look at how you manage your time. It will be time well spent.
- Learn to be realistic about your time. How much can you actually accomplish within a certain period of time? What is most important to do, and what can wait for another day?
- Make a list of things to be accomplished. Leave time for emergencies and unexpected events.
- Set priorities.
- Consider delegating or asking for help. Asking for help does not mean you are weak or incompetent.
- Schedule time to "stop and smell the flowers." We often forget to schedule time to take care of ourselves.

Module 11

Stress in Caring for Older People: Vignettes

1. Consuelo is concerned that she is not performing well at work, even though her clients and supervisor tell her that she is doing a good job. How can she reduce her stress?

a. Try hard to improve the quality of her work.

b. Look for a different job.

c. Spend more time thinking about her positive qualities and what she does well at work.

d. Go out and have a few beers.

2. Susan has been planning a vacation from work to spend some time with her family. At the last minute, her supervisor tells her that she cannot go at that time because the facility will be short-staffed. How should Susan respond to this stressful situation?

a. Accept her supervisor's decision and act as though there is nothing wrong.

b. Threaten to quit unless she is given the time off.

c. Tell her supervisor that she is upset and ask her to reschedule the vacation within the next month.

d. Go directly to the director to voice a complaint.

3. Rolanda has a full list of work to do at Mrs. Martin's house. Mrs. Martin asks if Rolanda could go to the grocery store to get her a carton of ice cream.

a. Tell Mrs. Martin that she will go as soon as she is finished with her work.

b. Drop what she is doing and leave immediately for the store.

c. Ignore the request.

d. Tell Mrs. Martin that she is sorry that she cannot go at this time but will buy Mrs. Martin's favorite flavor of ice cream when she does the shopping on her next visit.

4. Rosie works long hours, after which she is expected to go home to seemingly endless household chores. Her spouse and children are also busy and do not have time to help her. What should she do to get rid of some of this daily stress?

a. Work fewer hours.

b. Completely ignore the household chores and begin pampering herself.

c. Call a family meeting where she discusses her feelings and delegates chores to each member of the family.

d. Yell at her family, getting her anger off her chest.

Module 11

Relaxation Techniques for Caregivers

Deep-Breathing Exercises

Lie on the floor, with your head elevated slightly by a pillow. Your knees should be bent, with feet comfortably flat on the floor, about 8–12 inches apart. Place your left hand on your chest and right hand on your abdomen. Breathe in through your nose, taking in deep, even breaths to make your stomach rise. Your left hand should hardly move at all. Exhale through your mouth, whispering a sound like "aaaah." As you exhale, your jaw should be open slightly with mouth relaxed. Repeat, taking deep slow breaths for at least 5–10 minutes. Breathing should be slow, regular and relaxed.

Progressive Relaxation

Often you do not realize how tense your muscles become during a stressful situation. The following exercise will show you the contrast between muscle tension and relaxation.

- Sit quietly in a comfortable position.
- Close your eyes.
- Practice breathing (inhale through nose, expanding the stomach; exhale through nose or mouth, contract the stomach).
- Beginning with the right hand, tense muscles by making a tight fist, and concentrate on the tension.
- Hold for 3 seconds.
- Release the tension by uncurling your fingers and relaxing your hand. Concentrate on the relaxed state.
- Repeat tension-relaxation portion of the exercise.
- Continue the process using various muscle parts of the body.
- At various times during exercise, take a break, using the breathing exercise.
- Remember to tense and relax each muscle part twice.
- Concentrate on both the tension and relaxation.

Passive Relaxation

Repeat the steps above. Now try to relax every part of your body *without* first tensing your muscles.

Meditation and Imagery

Remove yourself from momentary stressors by visualizing a calm, peaceful scene. Focus your complete attention on a sound or image. This can reduce some of the physical effects of stress and help you feel calmer and more relaxed. Get in a comfortable position, close your eyes, and picture this:

> You are sitting on top of a grassy hill, overlooking the ocean. The sun is just beginning to set. It is comfortably warm as the sea breezes gently caress you. In the far distance, the water and horizon meet softly. The distinction of the two are blended into one mosaic. Notice how peaceful and content you feel. Carry your troubles out into the water. Release them and observe them float away with each passing wave. Stretch and exhale as you complete the exercise.

Stretching

An automatic physical response to stress is muscle tension. A simple, easy way to loosen tight muscles is to do stretching exercises. They only take a few minutes and can be done anywhere.

- Back stretch: While sitting, stretch forward, rest your body on your lap, and relax your head and neck. Hold for 1 minute, then press on your thighs to help yourself sit back up.
- Neck stretch: While standing or sitting, slowly rotate your head in a circle to the right without moving your shoulders. Then rotate to the left. Repeat five times on each side.
- Shoulder and arm stretch: Hold your hands together with fingers interlaced and stretch overhead with palms upward. Hold for 30 seconds, relax, and repeat five times.
- Passive back stretch: Lie on the floor with your legs on a chair. Relax, pressing your lower back onto the floor. Rest in this position for several minutes.
- Upper body stretch: With your feet a shoulder's width apart, reach overhead and stretch to the side. Try not to move your hips. Hold for 30 seconds; then switch sides.

References

Alexander, F., & Duff, R. (1988). Drinking in retirement communities. *Generations, 12*(4), 58–62.

American Psychiatric Association. (1994). *Desk reference to diagnostic criteria from DSM-IV*. Washington, DC: Author.

Beizer, J.L. (1984). Medications and the aging body: Alteration as a function of age. *Generations, 18*, 13–17.

Billig, N. (1987). *To be old and sad: Understanding depression in the elderly*. Lexington, MA: Lexington Books.

Birren, J.E., & Schaie, K.W. (Eds.). (1990). *Handbook of psychology of aging* (3rd ed.). San Diego: Academic Press.

Blanchard, K., & Johnson, S. (1983). *The one-minute manager*. New York: Berkley Books.

Blazer, D. (1990). *Emotional problems in later life*. New York: Springer.

Cooper, J.W. (1994). Drug-related problems in the elderly patient. *Generations, 18*, 19–27.

Fahey, C. (1983). Policy and ethical concerns regarding interventions with the acting-out elderly. In M.K. Aronson, R. Bennet, & B.J. Gurland (Eds.), *The acting out elderly* (pp. 73–78). New York: Haworth Press.

Goliszek, A. (1987). *Breaking the stress habit*. Winston-Salem, NC: Carolina Press.

Kubler-Ross, E. (1970). *On death and dying*. New York: Macmillan.

Lane, P. (1993). Using education techniques to teach—not to train—home care aides. *Caring Magazine, 12*(4), 51.

Maddox, G. (1988). Aging, drinking and alcohol abuse. *Generations, 12*(4), 14–16.

National Center for Health Statistics. (1992). *Facts about older Americans*. Washington, DC: Author.

National Institute on Aging. (1991). *What's your aging I.Q.?* Rockville, MD: Author.

National Institutes of Health Publication #94-3590 (1994). U.S. Department of Health and Human Services, Public Health Service, National Institutes of Health, Rockville, MD.

Petersen, D. (1988). Substance abuse, criminal behavior, and older people. *Generations, 12*(4), 63–67.

Richman, N., & Glantz, C. (1992a). *Sensory deficits and ways to help*. Unpublished manuscript. Riverwoods, IL: Rehabilitation Associates.

Richman, N., & Glantz, C. (1992b). *Sensory dysfunction exercise*. Unpublished manuscript. Riverwoods, IL: Rehabilitation Associates.

Richman, N., & Glantz, C. (1992). *101 ways to use capabilities*. Unpublished manuscript. Rehabilitation Associates, Riverwoods, IL.

Schmall, V.L., & Stiehl, R.E. (1990a). *The final course.* Corvallis: Oregon State University Extension Service.

Schmall, V.L., & Stiehl, R.E. (1990b). *Winter comforts.* Corvallis: Oregon State University Extension Service.

Scannell, E., & Newstrom, J. (1983). *More games trainers play.* New York: McGraw-Hill.

Sherman, D. (1994). Geriatric psychopharmacotherapy: Issues and concerns. *Generations, 18,* 34.

Simonson, W. (1994). Geriatric drug therapy: Who are the stakeholders? *Generations, 18,* 7–12.

Skeist, R.J. (1980). *To your good health! A practical guide for older Americans, their families, and friends.* Chicago: Chicago Review Press.

Sorensen, G. (1981). *The helping relationship: Ethical considerations in older persons and service providers.* New York: Human Sciences Press.

Totara, T. (1993). Understanding the nature and scope of domestic elder abuse with the use of state aggregate data: Summaries of the key findings of a national survey of state APS and aging agencies. *Journal of Elder Abuse and Neglect,* (5)4, 35–58.

Illinois Department of Public Health. *What everyone should know about AIDS.* (1983). Springfield, IL: Author.

Suggested Reading

ADULT LEARNING PRINCIPLES

Bibliography for teaching adults. (1993). *Caring Magazine, 12*(4), 52.

Banta, T.W. (Ed.). (1988). *Implementing outcomes assessment: Promise and perils.* San Francisco: Jossey-Bass.

Courtenay, B.C. (Ed.). (1986). *Helping older adults learn.* Washington, DC: American Association for Adult and Continuing Education.

Courtney, S. (1992). *Why adults learn: Towards a theory of participation in adult education.* New York: Routledge Publishers.

Cross, K.P. (1981). *Adults as learners.* San Francisco: Jossey-Bass.

Edwards, R., Sieminski, S., & Zeldin, D. (1993). *Adult learners, education, and training: A reader.* New York: Routledge Publishers.

Gueletter, D.G. (Ed.). (1986). *Using technology in adult education.* Washington, DC: American Association for Adult and Continuing Education.

Hayes, E. (Ed.). (1989). *Effective teaching styles.* San Francisco: Jossey-Bass.

Heimstra, R., & Sisco, B. (1990). *Individualizing instruction.* San Francisco: Jossey-Bass.

Korb, K., Azok, S., & Leutenberg, E. (1991). *Life management skills: Reproducible activity handouts created for facilitators.* Beachwood, OH: Wellness Reproductions, Inc.

Langerman, P.D. (Ed.). (1974). *You can be a successful teacher of adults.* Washington, DC: National Association for Public and Continuing Education.

Lewis, L.H. (Ed.). (1986). *Experiential and simulation techniques for teaching adults.* San Francisco: Jossey-Bass.

Lowman, J. (1984). *Mastering the techniques of teaching.* San Francisco: Jossey-Bass.

Merriam, S.B. (Ed.). (1986). *Being responsive to adult learners.* Washington, DC: American Association for Adult and Continuing Education.

Merriam, S.B., & Carrareia, R.S. (1991). *Learning in adulthood.* San Francisco: Jossey-Bass.

Mezirow, J. (1991). *Transformative dimensions of adult learning.* San Francisco: Jossey-Bass.

Mezirow, J. et al. (1990). *Fostering critical reflection in adulthood.* San Francisco: Jossey-Bass.

Mocker, D.W. (Ed.). (1986). *Teaching reading to adults.* Washington, DC: American Association for Adult and Continuing Education.

The National Eldercare Institute on Human Resources, Brookdale Center on Aging of Hunter College. *Using videos and visual aids: Tips for presenters.* New York: Author.

Remnet, V.L. (1989). *Understanding older adults: An experiential approach.* Lexington, MA: Lexington Books.

Rossman, M. H., & Rossman, M. E. (Eds.). (1990). *Applying adult development strategies.* San Francisco: Jossey-Bass.

Scannell, E., & Newstrom, J.W. (1981). *Games trainers play, experiential learning exercises.* New York: McGraw-Hill.

Scannell, E., & Newstrom, J.W. (1981). *More games trainers play, experiential learning exercises.* New York: McGraw-Hill.

Scannell, E., & Newstrom, J.W. (1981). *Still more games trainers play, experiential learning exercises.* New York: McGraw-Hill.

Sinnott, J. (Ed.). (1994). *Interdisciplinary handbook of adult lifespan learning.* Westport, CT: Greenwood Press.

Smith, R.M. (Ed.). (1983). *Helping adults learn how to learn.* San Francisco: Jossey-Bass.

Tuijnman, A.C., & van der Kamp, M. (Eds). (1992). *Learning across the lifespan: Theories, research and policies.* New York: Pergamon Press.

Ulmer, C. (1969). *Teaching the disadvantaged adult.* Washington, DC: National Association for Public and Continuing Education.

Vella, J.K. (1994). *Learning to listen, learning to teach: The power of dialogue in educating adults.* San Francisco: Jossey-Bass.

HOME HEALTH CARE

Handy, J., & Schuerman, C. (1994). *Challenges and innovations in homecare.* San Francisco: American Society on Aging.

Ory, M., & Duncker, A. (Eds.). (1992). *In-home care for older people: Health and supportive services.* Newbury Park, CA: Sage Publications.

Quinlan, A. (1988). *Chronic care workers.* Washington, DC: Older Women's League.

Romaine-Davis, A., Lenihan, A., & Shannon, M. (1992). *Home health care: An annotated bibliography.* New York: Greenwood Press.

Rowland, D., & Lyons, B. (Eds.). (1991). *Financing home care: Improving protection for disabled elderly people.* Baltimore: Johns Hopkins University Press.

AGING

Billig, N. (1992). *Older and wiser: Coping with expectations, challenges, and change in the later years.* New York: Lexington Books.

Fried, S., VanBooven, D., & MacQuarrie, C. (1993). *Older adulthood: Learning activities for understanding aging.* Baltimore: Health Professions Press.

Hendricks, J., & Hendricks, C.D. (1986). *Aging in mass society: Myths and realities* (3rd ed.). Boston: Little, Brown.

Hooyman, N.R., & Kujak, H.A. (1988). *Social gerontology: A multidisciplinary perspective.* Boston: Allyn & Bacon.

National Institute on Aging. *Age words: A glossary on health and aging.* Washington, DC: Author.

Russell, C. (1989). *Good news about aging.* New York: John Wiley & Sons.

Sorensen, G. (1981). *Older persons and service providers: An instructor's training manual.* New York: Human Sciences Press.

Remnet, V. (1989). *Understanding older adults: An experiential approach to learning.* Lexington, MA: Lexington Books.

Women of the Georgian Hotel. (1992). [Video]. (Distributed by Terra Nova Films, 9848 S. Winchester Avenue, Chicago, IL 60643.)

Additional Resources

The following organizations have catalogs of current resource materials on aging. The materials published include books, games, tapes, and kits on a wide-ranging body of subjects.

Bifolkal Productions, Inc., 809 Williamson Street, Madison, WI 53703

Elder Games, 11710 Hunter's Lane, Rockville, MD 20852

Golden Horizons, Virginia Darnell, P.O. Box 193, Sullivan, IL 61951

Potentials Development, 775 Main Street, Buffalo NY 14203

COMMUNICATION

Adler, R., & Rodman, G. (1985). *Understanding human communication.* New York: CBS College Publishing.

Atwater, E. (1992). *I hear you.* New York: Walker & Co.

Cox, B.J., & Waller, L. (1991). *Bridging the communication gap with the elderly.* Chicago: American Hospital Association.

Hyde, R. (1988). Facilitative communication skills training: Social support for elderly people. *Gerontologist, 28*(3), 418–420.

Pelsma, D., & Flanagan, M. (1986). Human relations training for the elderly. *Journal of Counseling and Development, 65(1),* 52–53.

DEPRESSION, SUICIDE, AND MENTAL ILLNESS

Billig, N. (1987). *To be old and sad: Understanding depression in the elderly.* Lexington, MA: Lexington Books.

Birren, J.E., Sloan, R.B., & Cohen, G.D. (Eds.). (1992). *Handbook of mental health and aging.* (2nd ed.). San Diego: Academic Press.

Blazer, D.G. (1990). *Emotional problems in later life.* New York: Springer.

Blazer, D.G. (1993). *Depression in later life.* St. Louis: Mosby/YearBook.

Butler, R., Lewis, M., & Sunderland, T. (1991). *Aging and mental health: Positive psychosocial and biomedical approaches.* (4th ed.). New York: Macmillan.

Characteristics of elderly suicide. (July 23, 1990). *The Brown University Long-Term Care Letter,* 2(14), 7(1).

Hinrichsen, G.A. (1990). *Mental health and older adults: Choices and challenges.* Santa Barbara, CA: ABC-CLIO, Inc.

Jeste, D., & Zisook, S. (Guest Eds.). (1988). Psychosis and depression in the elderly. *Psychiatric Clinics of North America, 11*(1).

Leenars, A.A., Maris, R., Macintosh, J., & Richman, J. (Eds.). (1992). *Suicide and the older adult.* New York: Guilford Press.

Starkstein, S., & Robinson, R. (1993). *Depression in neurologic disease.* Baltimore: Johns Hopkins University Press.

Suicidal seniors: Deadly serious. (February 9, 1991). *Science News, 139*(6), 92(1).

ALZHEIMER'S DISEASE AND OTHER DEMENTIAS

Alzheimer's Association, Chicago Area Chapter. (1988). *Home care with the Alzheimer's patient.* Skokie, IL (4709 Golf Road, Suite 1015).

Bauer, C. (1986). *When I grow too old to dream: A journal on Alzheimer's disease.* New York: Vantage Press.

Chavin, M. (1991). *The lost chord: Reaching the person with dementia through the power of music.* Mt. Airy, MD: ElderSong Publications.

Cohen, D., & Eisdorfer, C. (1986). *Loss of self: A family resource for the care of Alzheimer's disease and related disorders.* New York: Norton.

DeBolt, N., & Kastner, M.E. (1989). *I'm in here.* Torrington, WY (82240): Lutheran Health Systems (Goshen Care Systems, 536 E. 20th).

Edwards, A. (1994). *When memory fails: Helping the Alzheimer's and dementia patient.* New York: Plenum.

Feil, N. (1993). *The Validation breakthrough: Simple techniques for communicating with people with "Alzheimer's-Type Dementia."* Baltimore: Health Professions Press.

Freeman, S. (1990). *Activities and approaches for Alzheimer's.* Knoxville, TN: Whitfield Agency.

Guttman, R. (1991). *Adult day care for Alzheimer's patients: Impact on family caregivers.* New York: Garland Publishers.

Gwyther, L. (1985). *Care of Alzheimer's patients—A manual for nursing home staff.* Washington, DC: American Health Care Association.

Hamdy, R.C., Turnbull, J.M., Norman, L.K., & Lancaster, M.M. (Eds.). (1990). *Alzheimer's disease: A handbook for caregivers.* St. Louis: C.V. Mosby.

Hellen, C. (1992). *Alzheimer's disease: Activity-focused care.* Stoneham, MA: Andover Medical Publishers.

Huppert, F., Brayne, C., & O'Connor, D. (Eds.). (1994). *Dementia and normal aging.* New York: Cambridge University Press.

Lewis-Long, M. (1989). *Realistic Alzheimer's activities.* Amherst, NY: Potentials Development for Health and Aging Services.

Nissenboim, S., & Vroman, C. (1989). *Interaction by design.* St. Louis: Geri-Active Consultants.

Peckham, C.W. (1985). *Activities keep me going.* (Available from Otterbein Home, Lebanon, OH 45036.)

Rau, M. (1993). *Coping with communication challenges in Alzheimer's disease.* San Diego, CA: Singular Publishing Group.

Robinson, A. (1992). *Understanding difficult behaviors.* Ypsilanti, MI: Geriatric Education Center of Michigan.

Sheridan, C. (1987). *Failure free activities for Alzheimer's patients.* Oakland, CA: Cottage Books.

Terry, R., Katzman, R., & Bick, K. (Eds.). (1994). *Alzheimer's disease.* New York: Raven Press.

Wright, L. (1993). *Alzheimer's disease and marriage: An intimate account.* Newbury Park, CA: Sage Publications.

Zgola, J. (1987). *Doing things: A guide to programming activities for persons with Alzheimer's disease and related disorders.* Baltimore: Johns Hopkins University Press.

DEATH AND GRIEF

Bertman, S. (1991). *Facing death: Images, insights and interventions.* Bristol, PA: Taylor & Francis.

Callanan, M., & Kelley, P. (1992). *Final gifts: Understanding the special awareness, needs and communication of the dying.* New York: Poseidon Press.

Irish, D., Lundquist, K., & Nelson, V. (1993). *Ethnic variations in dying, death & grief: Diversity in universality.* Bristol, PA: Taylor & Francis.

Kastenbaum, R. (Ed.). (1994). *Death, society, and human experience.* Needham Heights, MA: Allyn & Bacon.

Knott, E., Ribar, M., Duson, B., & King, M. (1989). *Thanatopics: Activities and exercises for confronting death.* Lexington, MA: Lexington Books.

Kubler-Ross, E. (1970). *On death and dying.* New York: Macmillan.

Stroebe, M., Stroebe, W., & Hansson, R.O. (Eds.). (1993). *Handbook of bereavement.* New York: Cambridge University Press.

SUBSTANCE MISUSE AND ABUSE

Adams, S.L., & Waskel, S.A. (1993). Late onset alcoholism: Stress of structure. *Journal of Psychology, 127,* 329–34.

Ahronheim, J.C. (1992). *Handbook of prescribing medications for geriatric patients.* Boston: Little, Brown.

Alcohol and drugs: Abuse and misuse. (1990). *Generations, 12*(4).

Ascione, F. (1994). Medication compliance in the elderly. *Generations, 18*(2), 28–33.

Bloom, H.G., & Shlom, E. (1993). *Drug prescribing for the elderly.* New York: Raven Press.

Burke, M.M., & Walsh, M.B. (1992). *Gerontological nursing care of the frail elderly.* St. Louis: Mosby/YearBook.

Chastin, S. (1992). The accidental addict—Are you hooked on your prescriptions? *Modern Maturity,* February–March, 39–41.

Cooper, J.W. (1991). *Drug-related problems in geriatric nursing home patients.* Binghamton, NY: Haworth Press.

Cooper, J.W. (1993). *Community and nursing home drug monitoring guidelines—1993.* Watkinsville, GA: Consultant Press.

Ebersole, P. (1990). *Toward healthy aging: Human needs and nursing response* (3rd ed.). St. Louis: C.V. Mosby.

Forster, L.E. et al. (1993). Alcohol use and potential risk for alcohol-related adverse drug reactions among community-based elderly. *Journal of Community Health, 18,* 225–39.

Higbee, M.D. (1994). Consumer guidelines for using medications wisely. *Generations, 18*(2), 43–47.

Jennison, K. (1992). The impact of stressful life events and social support on drinking among older adults: A general population survey. *International Journal of Aging and Human Development, 35*(2), 99–123.

Lipton, H.L., & Lee, P.R. (1988). *Drugs and the Elderly: Clinical, social and policy perspectives.* Stanford, CA: Stanford University Press.

Mangion, D.M. (1992). Alcohol and acute medical admission of elderly people. *Age and Aging, 21,* 362–367.

Midanik, L.T. et al. (1992). Alcohol problems and sense of coherence among older adults. *Social Science and Medicine, 34*(1), 43–48.

Mulford, H.A., & Fitzgerald, J.L. (1992). Elderly vs. younger problem drinker profiles: Do they indicate a need for special programs for the elderly? *Journal of Studies of Alcohol, 53*, 601–610.

Opdycke, R.A.C.O. et al. (1992). A systematic approach to educating elderly patients about their medications. *Patient Education and Counseling, 19*, 43–60.

Pratt, C.C., Wilson, W., Benthin, A., & Schmall, V. (April, 1992). Alcohol problems and depression in later life: Development of two knowledge quizzes. *Gerontologist*, 175.

Robertson, N. (February–March, 1992). The intimate enemy—Will that friendly drink betray you?, *Modern Maturity*, 26–30.

Ruben, D. (1990). *The aging and drug effects: A planning manual for medication and alcohol abuse treatment in the elderly*. Jefferson, NC: McFarland & Co.

Schmall, V., & Stiehl, R.E. (1990). *Winter comforts: A workshop guide on how to identify and deal effectively with the older person who has a problem with alcohol*. Corvallis: Oregon State University.

Schonfeld, L. (1990). Older problem drinkers. Long term and late life onset abusers: What triggers their drinking? *Aging, 58*, 5–11.

Williamson, J., & Chopin, J.M. (1980). Adverse reactions to prescribed drugs in the elderly: A multicentre investigation. *Age and Ageing, 9*, 73–80.

Wolinsky, H. (Spring 1988). Combating America's 'other' drug problem. *Senior Care*.

ELDER ABUSE

A safer place. (1992). [Video]. (Distributed by The Illinois Department on Aging, 421 Capitol Avenue, Springfield, IL, 62701.)

Blakely, B.E. et al. (1993). Improving the responses of physicians to elder abuse and neglect: Contributions of a model program. *Journal of Gerontological Social Work, 19*(3, 4), 35–47.

Coyne, A.C. et al. (1993). The relationship between dementia and elder abuse. *American Journal of Psychiatry, 150*, 643–644.

Decalmer, P., & Glendenning, F. (1993). *The mistreatment of elderly people*. Newbury Park, CA: Sage Publications.

Elder abuse: Five case studies. (1991). [Video]. (Distributed by Terra Nova Films, 9848 S. Winchester Avenue, Chicago, IL 60642.)

Griffin, L.W. (March 1992). Abuse among African American elderly. *Journal of Family Violence*, 19–35.

Lachs, M.S. et al. (1994). A prospective community-based pilot study of risk factors for the investigation of elderly mistreatment. *Journal of the American Geriatric Society, 42*, 169–173.

Moon, A., & Williams, O. (1993). Perceptions of elder abuse and help-seeking patterns among African American, caucasian American, & Korean American elderly women. *Gerontologist, 33*(3), 386–395.

Paveza, G.J., Cohen, D., Eisdorfer, C., Freels, S., & Semla, T. (1992). Severe family violence and Alzheimer's disease: Prevalence and risk factors. *Gerontologist, 32*, 493–497.

Pillemer, K., & Hudson, B. (1993). A model abuse prevention program for nursing assistants. *Gerontologist, 33,* 128–131.

Pillemer, K., & Suitor, J.J. (1992). Violence and violent feelings: What causes them among family caregivers? *Journal of Gerontology, 47,* S165–S172.

Pritchard, J. (1992). *The abuse of elderly people: A handbook for professionals.* Bristol, PA: Taylor & Francis.

Responding to family violence. (A training resource for providers of home-based care. Available from Home Support Canada, 104-119 Ross Avenue, Ottawa, ON, Canada K1Y ON6.)

Steinmetz, S.K. (1990). Elder abuse: myth and reality. In T.H. Brubaker (Ed.), *Family relationships in later life.* (p. 193). Newbury Park, CA: Sage Publications.

Travalino, J. (June, 1993). Elder mistreatment: A call for help. *Patient Care,* 93–130.

Weith, M.E. (1994). Elder abuse: A national tragedy. *FBI Law Enforcement Bulletin, 63,* 24–26.

Wilson-Nolan, B.E., & Toone, C. (1993). Responding to family violence. *Caring Magazine, XII*(4), 32–35.

Wolf, R. (1994). What's new in elder abuse programming? Four bright ideas. *Gerontologist, 34*(1), 126–129.

Wolf, R.S. (1992). Making an issue of elder abuse. *Gerontologist, 32,* 427–429.

ETHICS IN THE CARE OF OLDER PEOPLE

Autonomy and long-term care. (1988). *Gerontologist, 28* (Suppl.)

Binstock, R., Post, S., & Whitehouse, P. (1992). *Dementia and aging: Ethics, values and policy choices.* Baltimore: Johns Hopkins University Press.

Christiansen, D. (1987). Ethical guidelines for assisting the elderly. *America,* 72–75.

Cohen, E.S. (1988). The elderly mystique: Constraints on the autonomy of the elderly with disabilities. *Gerontologist, 28,* 24–31.

Collopy, B., Dubler, N., & Zuckerman, C. (1990). The ethics of home care: Autonomy and accommodation. *Hastings Center Report, 20*(2), 1–16.

Jecker, N. (1991). *Aging and ethics: Philosophical problems in gerontology.* Clifton, NJ: Humana Press.

Kane, R.A., & Caplan, H.L. (1993). *Ethical conflict in the management of home care: The case manager's dilemma.* New York: Springer.

Kapp, M. (1992). *Ethical aspects of health care for the elderly: An annotated bibliography.* Westport, CT: Greenwood Press.

Logue, B. (1993). *Last rights: Death control and the elderly in America.* New York: Lexington Books.

Monagle, J., & Thomasma, D. (Eds.). (1994). *Health care ethics: Critical issues.* Gaithersburg, MD: Aspen Publishers.

National Association for Home Care. *Model bill of rights for clients and providers.* (Available from the National Association for Home Care, 519 C St., NE, Washington, DC 20002.)

Randall, D.A. (1989). Patient's rights & provider responsibility. *Pride Institute Journal of Long Term Home Health Care, 8*(2), 4–11.

Winslow, G., & Walters, J. (Eds.). (1993). *Facing limits: Ethics and health care for the elderly.* Boulder, CO: Westview Press.

STRESS MANAGEMENT

Benson, H., & Proctor, W. (1985). *Beyond the relaxation response.* New York: Berkley Publishing.

Bovysenko, J. (1987). *Minding the body, mending the mind.* Reading, MA: Addison-Wesley.

Chopra, D. (1994). *Ageless body, timeless mind.* New York: Crown.

Cousins, N. (1980). *Anatomy of an illness.* New York: Bantam Books.

Davis, M., & Eshelman, E.R. (1988). *Stress management: The relaxation and stress reduction workbook.* Oakland, CA: New Harbinger Publications.

Friedrich, J. (1994). Managing stress with nutrition and relaxation. *Let's Live, 6*(4), 14–22.

Goliszek, A. (1987). *Breaking the stress habit.* Winston-Salem, NC: Carolina Press.

Jaffe, D., & Scott, C. (1984). *From burnout to balance.* New York: McGraw-Hill.

Karr, K.L. (1993). *Taking care of me: How caregivers can effectively deal with stress.* Buffalo, NY: Prometheus Books.

Korb, E., Azok, S., & Leutenberg, E. (1991). *Life management skills: Reproducible activity handouts created for facilitators.* Beachwood, OH: Wellness Reproductions, Inc.

Panel, C. (1991). *The complete guide to stress management.* New York: Plenum.

Schaef, A.W. (1990). *Meditations for women who do too much.* San Francisco: Harper Collins.

Welch, I.D., & Medeiros, D.C. (1982). *Beyond burnout.* Englewood Cliffs, NJ: Prentice Hall.

Index

Page numbers followed by "f" indicate figures; page numbers followed by "t" indicate tables.

AA, *see* Alcoholics Anonymous
Abuse, 103
  alcohol, 91–102, 120
    chronic, 57*f*, 58
  elder, 103–113, 119–120
  medication, 78–84, 120
  substance, 120
Abusive behavior, 110, 111*f*
Acceptance, of death, 123, 125*f*, 126
Acceptance of Gifts activity, 122
Active Listening activity, 34–35
Activities
  leisure, 73–74, 74*f*
  normalization, 65
  task-oriented, 74–76
Activities of daily living, helping clients with, 72–73
Adult education
  calling upon life experience, 3
  open and accepting atmosphere for, 2–3
  principles of adult learning, 1–6
  student characteristics and needs, 2*t*
  teaching techniques, 3
  teaching tips, 4–5
Adults, *see* Older adults
Ageism, 7, 9
Aging, process of, normal, 7–24
  attitudes toward, 9, 10
  cardiovascular changes in, 21
  empathy for, 13–15
  gastrointestinal changes in, 22–23
  genitourinary changes in, 23
  hearing changes in, 18–19
  musculoskeletal changes in, 24
  neurological changes in, 24
  skin and nail changes in, 20
  stereotypes about, 8–13
  taste and smell changes in, 20
  vision changes in, 15–17
Agitation, 71
AIDS-related dementia, 57*f*, 58
Alcohol abuse, 91–102
  barriers to treatment, 93–95, 94*f*
  chronic, 57*f*, 58
  guidelines regarding, for caregivers, 120
  interventions and treatments for, 100, 101*f*
  in older adults, 92–101, 95, 95*f*
  symptoms of, 98–99, 98*f*
Alcohol withdrawal symptoms, 92, 97
Alcoholics Anonymous (AA), 100
Alcoholism, 91
  chronic, 95
  early-onset, 91, 95–96
  facts about, 93*f*
  late-onset, 92, 95–96, 100–101
  reactive, 96
  risks for older adults, 96–97, 97*f*
Alzheimer's disease, 56*f*, 58–59
  attitudes toward, 12
  diagnosis of, 59
  stages and characteristics of, 63*t*–64*t*
Americans, older, facts about, 8*f*
Anger, 125*f*, 126

Anxiety, 71
Apathy, 70
Attitudes Toward Aging activity, 9

Bargaining, 123, 125*f*, 126
Barriers to communication, *see* Communication
Behavior
  abusive, 110, 111*f*
  active listening, 33, 34*f*
  associated with dementia, 70–72
  difficult, 43–46, 66, 70
    causes of, 66
    dealing with, 70
    depression as cause, 43–46
  ethical, regarding acceptance of money and gifts, 122, 122*f*
  inappropriate social or sexual, 71
Behavior problems, 68–70
  case studies, 69–70
  causes and triggers of, 68–69, 69*f*
Beliefs About Alcohol Problems activity, 92
Binswanger's disease, 58
Blackboards, as visual aid, 3
Brain, 59–63
  damage to, from Alzheimer's disease, 60–62
  frontal lobe, 59, 60*f*, 61
  information transmission in, 61
  occipital lobe, 60, 60*f*
  parietal lobe, 60, 60*f*
  segments of, 59–60, 60*f*
  temporal lobe, 59, 60*f*
Burnout, in care providers, 27, 131, 134

Cardiovascular changes in aging, 21*t*
Care providers
  looking at self, 135
  protecting, 112–113
  role of, 101–102, 117–118
  stress management for, 131–139
  taking care of self, 50–51
Changing the subject, in listening, 30, 32*f*
Closed-ended questions, 32*f*
Code of ethics, 116–117
Code of Ethics activity, 119
Commands, breaking down, 72
Communication, 25
  barriers to, 32*f*
  effective, 25–35
  message delivery, 29
  nonverbal, 29, 34*f*
  process of, 26, 26*f*
  putting thoughts into words, 28–29
  sending clear messages, 26–28
  talking, 32*f*
  techniques to use with clients who have hearing loss, 31*f*
  techniques to use with persons who have dementia, 67–68, 67*f*
  in workplace, 26
Communication problems, 66, 67*f*
Communication Vignette activity, 31–33
Confidentiality, 118
Confidentiality Case Studies activity, 118
The Confused Mind–What Is It Like? activity, 62
Confused older adults
  behavior problems in, 68–70
  caring for, 65–76
  causes of difficult behavior in, 66
  communication problems in, 66–68
  dementia, behaviors associated with, 70–72
Coping, 131, 135
Cues, 72, 73
  hand-over-hand, 73
  physical, 73
  verbal, 73
  visual, 73

Death and dying, 123–130
  acceptance of, 123, 125*f*, 126
  grief and, 124
    stages of, 124–126
  needs of dying people, 128–129
  religion, role of in, 129–130

responses to, 127
talking about, 129–130
Dehydration, 56*f*
Delirium tremens (DTs), 97
Dementia(s), 40–42
AIDS-related, 57*f*, 58
behavior problems in people with, 68–69, 69*f*
behaviors associated with, 70–72
causes of, 56*f*–57*f*
communication problems of people with, 66, 67*f*
definition of, 53, 55
leisure activities for clients with, 73
multi-infarct, 53, 57*f*, 58
Role Play activity, 68
symptoms of, 54–55
techniques for communicating with people with, 67*f*, 67–68
types of, 55–59
understanding, 53–64
ways to use remaining capabilities of people with, 75*f*–76*f*
Denial, 123, 125, 125*f*
Depressed persons
helping, 47*f*, 50–51
observation of, 41*f*, 41–42
subjects to talk about with, 44, 44*f*
Depression, 37–52, 56*f*, 70
cause of difficult behavior, 43–46
causes of, 42
definition of, 37, 38
versus dementia, 40–42
physical and visual clues, 41*f*, 41–42
prelude to suicide, 46–48
signs and symptoms of, 38–39, 39*t*, 40–41
as stage of grief, 125*f*, 126
treatment for, 42–43
types of, 38
untreated, 43
Depression Case Study activity, 42
Disapproval, showing, in listening, 32*f*
Discussion, small group, 4
Diseases, induced by stress, 132, 132*f*
"Doctor hopping," 80, 80*t*
Drugs, *see* Medication
DTs, *see* Delirium tremens
Dying, *see* Death and dying
Dysfunctional abusers, 103

Early-onset alcoholism, 91, 95–96
Education, *see* Adult education
Effective Communication activity, 89
Elder abuse, 103–113
available interventions for, 111–112
ethical issues, 119–120
guidelines for, 120
types of, 105, 105*f*, 106*t*
victims and abusers, characteristics of, 106–108, 107*f*, 108*t*, 109*f*
Elderly, *see* Older adults
Empathy, 7, 13–24, 37
Enabling, 91
Ethics, 115, 116
acceptance of money and gifts, 122, 122*f*
code of, 116–117
Exploitation, financial, *see* Financial exploitation

Facts on Aging activity, 10–13
False reassurance, 123
Family medical history, 59
Feedback, positive, 28
"Fight or flight" response, 133
Filtering, 127–128
Financial exploitation, 103, 105, 106*f*
indicators of, 110–111, 111*f*
Flip charts, as visual aid, 3
Focusing on the Client activity, 45

Gastrointestinal changes in aging, 22*t*–23*t*
Genitourinary changes in aging, 23*t*
Gifts, for care providers
acceptance of, 122
ethical behavior regarding, 122, 122*f*
guidelines regarding, 122
Grief, 56*f*
normal, 125–128
stages of, 125*f*, 125–126

Group discussion, 4
Guess My Line activity, 66

Hallucinations, 71
Handouts, as visual aid, 4
Hand-over-hand cues, 73
Hangovers, 97, 98–99
Hearing loss
  techniques to improve communication with clients with, 31*f*
  ways to help, 18*t*–19*t*
Hippocampus, 60, 60*f*
Home, wanting to go, and dementia, 71–72

"I Know" activity, 50–51, 51*t*–52*t*
Infection, 56*f*
Information, asking for more, in active listening, 34*f*, 35
In-service, preparation tasks for, 6*f*
Invalidation, 25
Is This Elder Abuse? activity, 104
Is This a Risky Situation? activity, 113
Isolation, 123, 125, 125*f*

Job responsibility, 119
Judgment, passing, 32*f*

Korsakoff's syndrome, 57*f*, 58, 96

Laboratory tests, *see* Tests
Late-onset alcoholism, 92, 95–96, 100–101
Learning, adult
  calling upon life experience, 3
  principles of, 1–6
Leisure activities
  for clients with dementia, 73
  purposes of, 74*f*
  value of, 73–74
Listening
  active, 25, 33, 34*f*
  effective skills for, 33, 33*f*
  passive, 25, 30

Measuring Coping Strategies activity, 135
Medical histories, 59
Medication
  and older adults, 78–84
    addiction in, 83
    errors and, 78
    hospitalization of, 78
    noncompliance and, 80, 82–83
    polypharmacy, 80
    regimens, complicated, 81
    self-medicating, 80
    sharing, 81–82
    side effects in, 81, 83
  psychotropic, 77
Medication abuse
  guidelines regarding, 120
  how to help, 88*f*
  prevention of, 87–90
  reasons for, 80, 80*t*
  signs and symptoms of, 85, 85*f*
Medication chart, 81, 82*f*
Medication problems, 56*f*
Medication use, abbreviations for, 87–88
Medication Use Quiz activity, 79
Memory loss, symptoms of, 54, 55*f*
Messages, in effective communication
  advice, giving, 31, 32*f*
  delivery, 26–28, 29
  receiving, 30–31
MID, *see* Multi-infarct dementia
Misuse, 77, *see also* Alcohol abuse; Medication abuse
Misuse Or Not? activity, 86–87
Money and gifts
  acceptance of, 122
  ethical behavior regarding, 122, 122*f*
  guidelines regarding, 122
  see also Ethics
Morals, 115, 116–117
Multi-infarct dementia (MID), 53, 57*f*, 58
Musculoskeletal changes in aging, 24*t*

Nail changes in aging, 21*t*
Needs, of terminally ill people, 128–129
Neglect, 103, 105, 106*f*
Nerve cells, 60, 61*f*
Neurological changes in aging, 24*t*
Neurological exams, *see* Tests
Noncompliance, 77, 80*t*, 81, 82–83
Nonjudgmental attitude, toward older people, 25, 101
Normalization activities, 65
Nostalgia, 74
Nutritional deficits, 56*f*

Older adults
  alcohol abuse in, 92–101, 95*f*, 97*f*
  confused, 65–76
  medication and, 78–84
  sexuality in, 120–121
  stereotypes about, 8–13
  suicide and, 48–49
  untreated depression in, 43
Older Americans, facts about, 8*f*
Origins of Ethics activity, 116
Osteoporosis, 7
Outside support, 136
Overhead projectors, as visual aid, 3

Paranoia, 71
Paraphrasing, 25, 33, 34*f*
Parkinson's disease, 57*f*, 58
Passive listening, 25, 30
Physical abuse, 109–111, 110*f*
Physical condition, in stress relief, 137–138
Physical cues, 73
Physical disease, 56*f*
Physical exam, *see* Tests
Platitudes, 25, 32*f*
Polypharmacy, 77, 80, 80*t*
Positive feedback, 28
Positive Feedback activity, 28
Practice sessions, in adult education, 4
Preparation tasks, for in-services, 6*f*
Psychiatric tests, *see* Tests
Psychological condition, in stress relief, 137–138
Psychological tests, *see* Tests
Psychotropic medications, *see* Medications

Questions
  closed-ended (yes/no), 32*f*
  for "I Know" game, 51*t*–52*t*
  repeated, 71
  "why," 32*f*

Radiologic tests, *see* Tests
Reassurance, false, 123
Reflecting, 34*f*, 35
Relaxation techniques, 137, 137*f*–138*f*
Religion, role in death and dying, 129–130
Reminiscence, 74
Reminiscing activity, 124
Repetition, in dementia, 71, 72
Respiratory changes in aging, 21*t*
Responses to Dying activity, 127
Restating, 25, 33
Restlessness, in dementia, 71
Role playing, in adult education, 4

Self-Care Inventory activity, 135–136
Self-esteem, 135
Self-medication, 80, 80*t*
Senility, 53, 54–55
Sensory deficit charts, 14, 15*t*–24*t*
Sensory Dysfunction Exercise activity, 13–14
Sensory problems, 56*f*
Sexual behavior, inappropriate, 71
Sexuality, 120–121
  guidelines regarding, 121
  myths and facts regarding, 121*f*
Sexuality in Older People activity, 121
Skills, for effective listening, 33, 33*f*
Skin changes in aging, 21*t*
Small group discussion, 4
Smell changes in aging, 20*t*
Social behavior, inappropriate, 71

Special Needs of Terminally Ill People and Their Families activity, 128
Stereotypes, 7, 8–13
Stereotypes of Aging activity, 9–10
Stress, 37, 56*f*
  definition of, 131
  diseases induced by, 132, 132*f*
  elements of, 132–134
  management of, 50–51, 134–135
  mediators of, 132, 133–134
  signs of, 133, 134*t*
  situations, 139
Stress Monitoring activity, 50
Stress reactions, 132, 133, 133*f*
Stressors, 132
Students, adult, 2*t*
Subject, changing the, and effective listening, 30, 32*f*
Substance abuse, 120
Suicide, 37
  depression as prelude to, 46–48
  and older people, 48–49
  risk of, 37–52
  warning signs of, 48*f*, 48–49
Suicide-prevention policy, model, 49*f*
Sundowning, 69, 71
Support, outside, 136
Suspicion, in dementia, 71

Take Your Medicine! activity, 84
Task analysis, 65, 72
Task Analysis activity, 72
Task-oriented activities, 74–76
Taste changes in aging, 20*t*
Teaching techniques, in adult education, 3
Teaching tips, in adult education, 4–5
Tearing a Sheet of Paper activity, 29
Tense Situations activity, 139
Terminally ill people, special needs of, 128–129
Test Your Observation and Reporting Skills activity, 27–28
Tests
  laboratory, 59
  neurological, 59
  psychiatric, 59
  psychological, 59
  radiologic, 59
Time management, 136*f*, 136–138
"Tip of the tongue" phenomenon, 54, 66

Use Or Abuse? activity, 99–100

Values, 115, 116
Values Clarification Exercise activity, 117
Verbal cues, 73
Videotape, as visual aid, 3–4
Vision changes in aging, 15*t*–17*t*
Visual aids, in adult education, *see specific types*
Visual cues, 73

Wandering, in dementia, 70–71
Ways of Communicating activity, 30
"Why" questions, 32*f*
Withdrawal, 70
  from alcohol, 92, 97
Word Meaning activity, 28–29
Words, putting thoughts into, as communication technique, 28–29
Workplace communication, 26